Walter Dandy: The Personal Side of a Premier Neurosurgeon

MARY ELLEN DANDY MARMADUKE

Editors:

Issam A. Awad, M.D.
Edward R. Laws, Jr., M.D.

Sponsored by
The Congress of Neurological Surgeons
2002

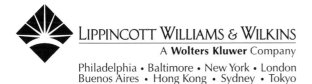

LIPPINCOTT WILLIAMS & WILKINS
A **Wolters Kluwer** Company

Philadelphia • Baltimore • New York • London
Buenos Aires • Hong Kong • Sydney • Tokyo

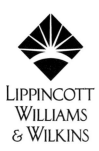

LIPPINCOTT
WILLIAMS
& WILKINS

Printed in the United States of America
(ISBN 0-7817-4237-4)

Walter Dandy: The Personal Side of a Premier Neurosurgeon

MARY ELLEN DANDY MARMADUKE

ISSAM A. AWAD, M.D., M.S.C, F.A.C.S.

The Ogsbury-Kindt Professor and Chairman
Department of Neurosurgery
University of Colorado School of Medicine
Denver, Colorado

EDWARD LAWS, JR., M.D., F.A.C.S.

Professor of Neurosurgery and Medicine
Department of Neurological Surgery
University of Virginia
Health Sciences Center
Charlottesville, Virginia

Sponsored by
The Congress of Neurological Surgeons
2002

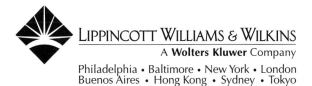

LIPPINCOTT WILLIAMS & WILKINS
A **Wolters Kluwer** Company
Philadelphia • Baltimore • New York • London
Buenos Aires • Hong Kong • Sydney • Tokyo

This book is dedicated to the members of Walter Dandy's family and the larger family of neurosurgeons who follow his example as a surgeon and clinician.

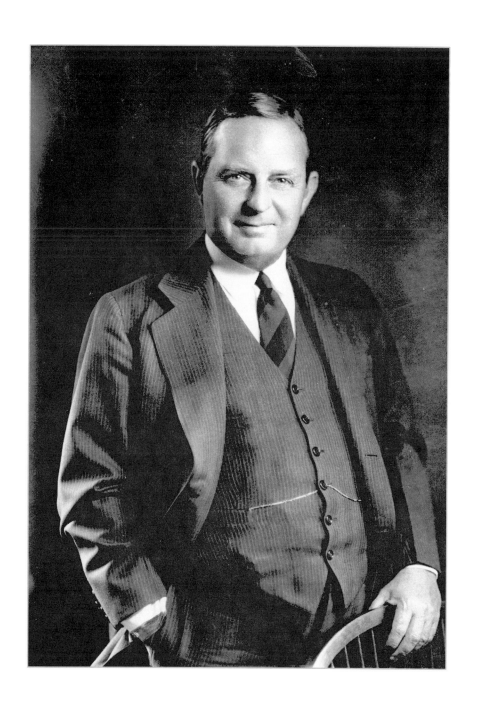

Walter E. Dandy, M.D.
1886–1946

$\mathscr{P}$reface

In every generation there are those with exceptional ability, whose intellectual or creative achievements gain distinction among their peers. Such premier leaders often exhibit extraordinary talent, a unique skill, and they exert a lasting influence on their field of endeavor. There is always a personal side to such genius; this side is more often gentle, and more vulnerable than the public persona. Walter E. Dandy, a giant figure in neurosurgery, was no exception. Rising from humble roots, he made his impact in a world of elitism and grand traditions at the Johns Hopkins Medical School. His early streaks of ambition, his mentorship under and later rivalry with Harvey Cushing, and the many accomplishments that were his own, have been widely studied. But these treatises did not do justice to Dr. Dandy's personal and private side, his vulnerability, his fondness, his generosity. These highly personal qualities were best shown to and most known by his family.

In countless special photographs, sorted and arranged with personal legends and anecdotes, Dr. Dandy's daughter, Mary Ellen Marmaduke, shares intimate family perspectives on this extraordinary man. New light is shed on the personal side of this premier neurosurgeon. This material had been assembled as a family album so that the Dandy grandchildren and great-grandchildren could cherish Dr. Dandy's memory. It was first brought to Dr. Awad's attention by Edward R. Laws, Jr., a close friend of the Dandy family, an admirer of his legacy, and a former president of the Congress of Neurological Surgeons (CNS). It became evident that this material ought to be shared with Dr. Dandy's larger family, the practicing neurosurgeons who have been so influenced by his legacy. A planning meeting was held in Denver, Colorado in June 2001. Ms. Marmaduke attended and presented a splendid lecture on "the private side of Walter Dandy as seen by his family" to a gathering of neurosurgeons from the University of Colorado and the Front Range communities. The idea for publication of this book under the sponsorship of the CNS was born.

That same month, the CNS Executive Committee warmly endorsed the publication of this book, and also the creation of a special archival website for Dr. Dandy's personal correspondence with his family from 1903 through 1946, along with a powerful search engine, at www.neurosurgery.org/CNS/Dandy/. As CNS president, Dr. Awad had the honor of formally announcing the CNS sponsorship of these projects at the 51st Annual meeting in San Diego in September 2001.

In the subsequent months, this material was carefully organized by Ms. Marmaduke, with thoughtful input from the other Dandy children, Kitty Dandy Gladstone, Margaret Dandy Gontrum, and Walter E. Dandy, Jr. Each added his or her personal reflections, memories, and anecdotes, as only devoted children can. The book was organized in five sections, reflecting Dr. Dandy's origins and early life, the making of a surgeon, his marriage, family and career, his passion for living, and his lasting legacy. The sections were edited with the love and admiration of privileged heirs by Drs. Awad and Laws. Additionally, they sought the insightful comments of a number of leading neurosurgeons who had unique perspectives and scholarly knowledge of Walter Dandy.

We were personally touched with grace and glory for the privilege of helping to catalyze the fruition of this unique publication. On behalf of the CNS, we express the deepest gratitude of the neurosurgeons of America and the world to the Dandy family for their generosity and consideration in sharing this very private material. Particular affection and warm friendship are reserved for Mary Ellen Marmaduke, acknowledging her thoughtful and persistent stewardship and guidance through the task of conceptualizing and executing this publication. We are grateful that the CNS has the unique privilege of helping preserve and publicize a special work of scholarship related to the Dandy legacy. We thank the editorial staff at Lippincott, Willliams, and Wilkins for their professionalism and thoughtful approach to every step of publication.

The CNS is grateful to the Dandy family and proud to sponsor the publication of this unique monograph as a gift to neurosurgeons of the world. This informative material befits the educational mission of the CNS. May this work enlighten future scholars and students of neurological surgery about the personal and human qualities that are so essential to premier leadership.

Issam A. Awad, MD, FACS
51st President
Congress of Neurological Surgeons
Denver, CO

Edward R. Laws, MD, FACS
34th President
Congress of Neurological Surgeons
Charlottesville, VA

$\mathscr{I}$ntroduction

I began this book to give my children, grandchildren, and their cousins a better understanding of my father, Walter Dandy. Because he died in 1946, before they were born, they knew him mainly through the stories my mother would recount about him. When she died in 1996, I felt a need to record his life story for them. I wanted these younger generations to know more about his warmth, humor, and enthusiasm for life. I wanted them to understand his contributions to medicine and to see him in the context of his own family and the times in which he lived. William Fox's biography, *Dandy of Johns Hopkins,* was rich in details of my father's life and career, but naturally Fox was not able to present the personal perspective that only Dandy's children could provide. With that in mind, I started this book in 1997.

My first task was to collect as many photographs of my father as possible. My brother, Walter, and sisters, Kitty and Maggie, delved into their boxes of pictures. Most of the family pictures had been taken and preserved by our mother, Sadie. Photographs were also added from the collections of the Alan Mason Chesney Archives at Johns Hopkins Medical Institutions.

For the accompanying text, I selected materials from a variety of sources. (See Bibliography, Appendix D). To present my father's career, I drew from articles by his contemporaries and those that followed him. In recent years, a number of insightful articles have been written by neurosurgeons who gave a historical perspective on his career. My father's letters gave unique insight into his personality, his relationships, and his world. Non-surgical perspectives were found in accounts of lay people, including newspaper articles from his hometown newspaper. Some may be legend, some fact; the reader can filter out a view of this colorful and interesting man.

This has been a family project. Each of my siblings contributed photographs, recollections, and advice. Kitty had previously collected and edited more than 200 letters exchanged between our father and his parents during the years between 1903-1914. Those letters gave day-to-day accounts of his early career. Maggie, a talented writer, was the first editor of this book. She took early drafts and made them come alive. Walter provided all sorts of help with his recollections of the past, articles from the Hopkins presses, and in-depth knowledge of our father's career. In addition, my daughters, Susan, Maggie, and Polly provided support, assorted editing, and assistance in deciphering the later series of letters. I give thanks to my good friends who patiently listened to my recounting of the saga of putting this book together.

The book entered a new phase in the spring of 2001. Ed Laws and I gave a joint presentation about my father at a conference we were both attending in Oregon. At that conference, I showed him an early draft of this book. He showed it to Issam Awad, who was President of the Congress of Neurological Surgeons at the time. Issam gained permission for the Congress to publish the book. He and Ed undertook to edit this version for the larger neurosurgical family. Throughout the process, they were both astute editors and unflagging supporters. Our trio worked together with remarkable trust and respect - rare qualities for a first-time team.

I sent the original version to three senior neurosurgeons: Hugo Rizzoli, George Hayes, and Harold Paxton. Hugo Rizzoli had been one of my father's last residents and a member of the original "Brain Team." George Hayes had known my father briefly during a rotation on the Brain Team during his surgical residency. Harold Paxton, as a medical student at Hopkins, had watched my father operate in his last years. Each made thoughtful comments. Kim Burchiel and Ed Neuwelt at OHSU and Issam in Denver gave me opportunities to make presentations about my father's life to colleagues whose questions and comments helped shape the book.

As we planned the book, Issam sought commentaries from neurosurgeons who had particular professional connections with Walter Dandy: John Oro from the University of Missouri Medical School, and Don Long and Henry Brem from Hopkins. Rafael Tamargo worked with Henry Brem on his piece. Ed Laws and Issam also agreed to write commentaries. Their perspectives greatly enrich the book.

There were other contributions by neurosurgeons. John Oro provided photographs of my father's hometown of Sedalia, Missouri, as well as the University of Missouri during my father's time there. As the book took shape, John did further research at the Historical Society in Columbia to answer some of my questions about those early years. The book includes observations taken from articles by various neurosurgeons, including Don Long, in particular. Henry Brem, Dandy Visiting Professor at Hopkins in 1995, asked questions about my father as a parent, making me aware that perhaps other neurosurgeons might be interested in a personal view of him. Peter Jannetta's generous establishment of the Walter Dandy Professorship in Pittsburgh in 1992 makes him a special member of the team. Without each and every member of the new "Brain Team", this book would not have been possible.

I have tremendous gratitude to Nancy MacCall and Marjorie Kehoe and their colleagues at the Alan Mason Chesney Archives at Johns Hopkins Medical Institutions for their assistance in all stages of the book. They were especially helpful in the early phases of my research in Baltimore. They guided me through the Dandy Collection, taught me about scanning, and allowed me to peruse the boxes of artifacts, including scrapbooks kept by my grandparents of my father's developing career, assorted clippings, photographs, the headlight my father designed, and his life mask. The editors at Lippincott Williams and Wilkins shepherded me through the editing and publishing process. With the 200 photographs and drawings, this was an intricate production.

Last, but not least, I am indebted to my "technical team" of electronic cohorts: computer and internet, scanner and other peripherals, without which this project could never had been completed in my lifetime. E-mail allowed me track my busy colleagues in this effort and allowed them to respond - whether in China, Europe, or wherever.

I hope as you read this book, Walter Dandy will become, for you, the vibrant personality I knew and loved. On behalf of my family, I want to express our appreciation to the Congress of Neurological Surgeons for publishing this perspective of Walter Dandy for the larger neurosurgical family.

Mary Ellen Dandy Marmaduke
Portland, Oregon
June 2002

Contents

CHAPTER 1

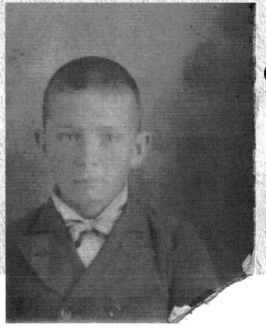

Origins and Early Life: 1886–1907

Walter Dandy as a schoolboy in Sedalia, 1894.

CHAPTER 1 OUTLINE

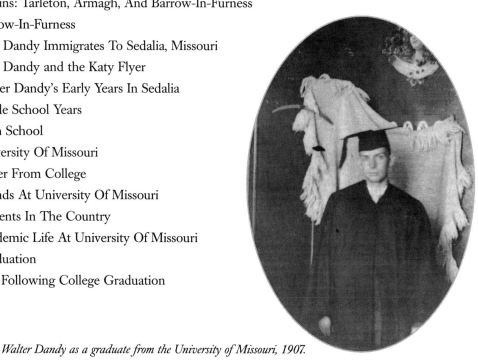

Walter Dandy as a graduate from the University of Missouri, 1907.

1

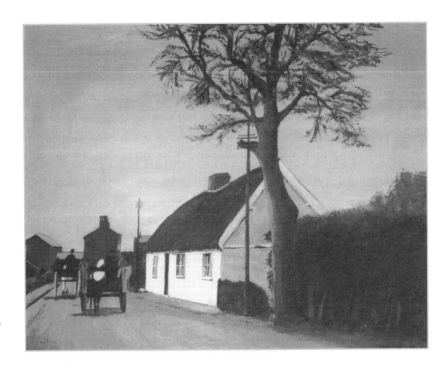

FIGURE 1.1
John Dandy's
family home in
Lancashire
County, England.

ORIGINS: TARLETON, ARMAGH, AND BARROW-IN-FURNESS

Walter Dandy's father, John Dandy, was born in 1856, in the small farming town of Tarleton in the County of Lancashire, in northwestern England (Figure 1.1). John and his family lived in this thatched roof cottage throughout his childhood.[1]

Times were hard for the Dandy family and others in northern England. John left school in the third grade to do farm work to help support the family. In 1870, at the age of fourteen, John, his mother, and his sister Nanny moved to the port city of Barrow-in-Furness to find work. After working in a steel mill, John moved on to a job as a foreman for the Furness Railroad.

Walter's mother, Rachel Kilpatrick, was born in 1861 in Bally Lane, a small farming community near the town of Armagh, in County Armagh, in northern Ireland (Figure 1.2). After graduating from high school, Rachel left the farm and crossed the Irish Sea to Barrow-in-Furness to find work as a seamstress (Figure 1.3).

BARROW-IN-FURNESS

John and Rachel met in 1881. John reported that he "fell in love with her at first sight."[2]

Many years later, John remembered the lovely lanes around Barrow "where Mama and I used to court," and "during my stay in England, I had many nice walks and talks with her."[3] He told his grandchildren years later that he had admired her lovely brown hair.

Barrow was a bustling port on the Irish Sea (Figure 1.4[4]). The town developed in the early nineteenth century when iron was discovered nearby. Jobs in shipping, iron and steel works, and railroads at first drew many workers, but an economic depression hit the area in the early 1880s. Many were emigrating in search of better working conditions.

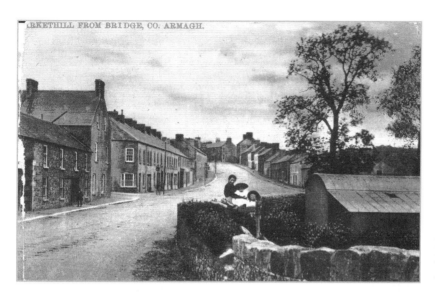

FIGURE 1.2
Rachel Kilpatrick Dandy was born near the town of Armagh, in Northern Ireland. This postcard was written in 1911.

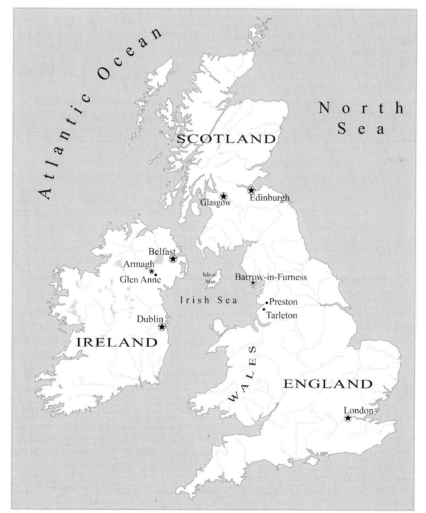

FIGURE 1.3
Map showing Tarleton, Armagh, and Barrow.

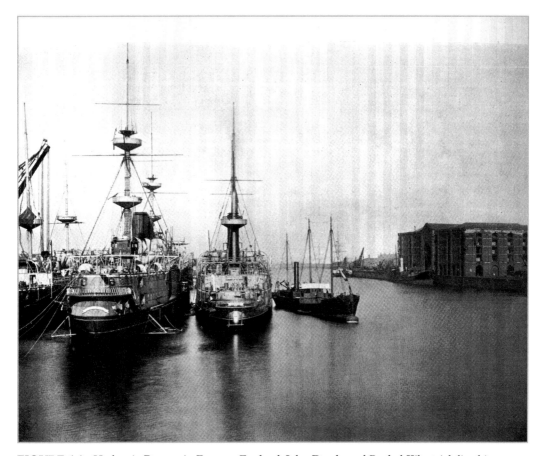

FIGURE 1.4   Harbor in Barrow-in-Furness, England. John Dandy and Rachel Kilpatrick lived in Barrow. This photo is from a book they apparently purchased in England during the period from 1911–1914.

John could not afford the passage to Australia or New Zealand, and turned down an offer to work on the "Cape to Cairo Railroad" in Africa. This railroad was proposed by Cecil Rhodes in 1881, but was never constructed. When Robert Battersby, a railroad friend from Barrow, wrote from Sedalia, Missouri, to describe the fine job opportunities in the rapidly developing railroads in America, John decided to emigrate to the United States. Rachel agreed to join him there when he found work.

John Dandy Immigrates to Sedalia, Missouri

John Dandy reached Sedalia in 1883 (Figure 1.5). There he joined his friend Robert Battersby, who had settled there with his wife, Magdalena. Like John, the Battersbys had been members of the Plymouth Brethren Church in England. Later their children, Stanley and Polly, also became lifelong friends of the Dandys.

The town of Sedalia (Figure 1.6), located between St. Louis and Kansas City, was founded in 1860 by General George G. Smith of the Pacific Railroad (later the Missouri Pacific ("MOPAC")). At the time of the Civil War, the area around Sedalia was home to

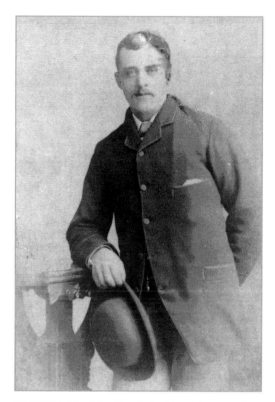

FIGURE 1.5   John Dandy in 1883. Photograph taken in Sedalia after he came from England.

many wealthy slave owners. Like the rest of Missouri, it supplied soldiers to both the Union and Confederate armies. After the Civil War, railroad lines multiplied in the West. Sedalia grew rapidly with connecting lines in all directions. As traffic increased along the lines, Sedalia became a railroad hub with the largest shops west of the Mississippi.[5] Trains passing through Sedalia carried settlers from the East Coast and immigrants from Europe in their search for cheap land, work, and adventure—the Westward Movement.

In 1866, the Missouri, Kansas, and Texas Railroad (MK&T) began construction on its Missouri line originating in Sedalia. The line extended into southeast Kansas and joined the Kansas line[6] to cross Indian Territory (now Oklahoma) and over the Red River into Texas. The first MK&T train arrived in Denison, Texas in 1872, eleven years before John Dandy was to come to Sedalia.

The census of 1890 listed Sedalia's population as 15,000. It was "known for the beauty and finished condition of its streets and avenues."[7]

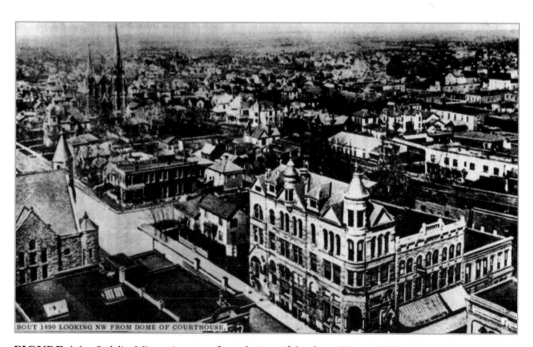

FIGURE 1.6   Sedalia, Missouri as seen from the top of the Court House, 1899.

JOHN DANDY AND THE KATY FLYER

When John Dandy arrived in Sedalia in 1883, he was hired as a fireman on MK&T. Eventually John became an engineer of the "Katy Flyer" (Figure 1.7). The fine record of this particular train earned it the epithet of "crack" train.

Railroading through the wild stretches of land between Missouri and Texas was a dangerous occupation in those days. Ambushes by train robbers were frequent: "Katy trains were derailed, looted, held up regularly along the lonely line from the early [eighteen] seventies until well into the present century."[8] Despite the difficult conditions and his family's concern for his safety, John Dandy worked on the Katy until his retirement in 1911.

WALTER DANDY'S EARLY YEARS IN SEDALIA

In 1885, Rachel sailed to New York and traveled by train to St. Louis. She and John were married the evening of her arrival, May 23, 1885. They traveled to Sedalia to set up housekeeping. Walter was born the following year. Years later, John Dandy wrote: "My son, Walter Edward, was born April 6, 1886 in Sedalia, and his mother adored him (Figure 1.9). He was quite a companion for her as I was away working on the R.R. and she never seemed lonesome after he was born."[9] A Sedalia surgeon, responding to the lore about Walter Edward Dandy, speculated many years later: "Rachel was remembered as the neighborhood's most meticulous housekeeper and best cook, and it is probably from his mother that Walter acquired his respect for excellence and superior standards."[10]

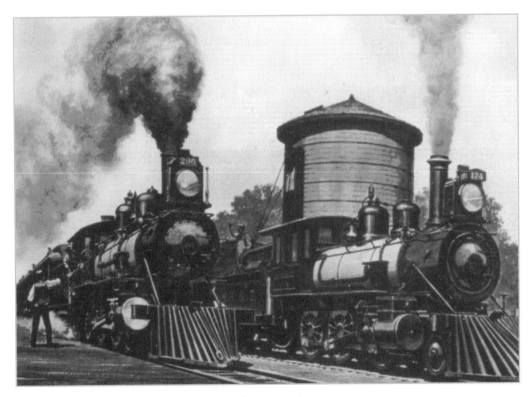

FIGURE 1.7 John Dandy's train, The Katy Flyer.

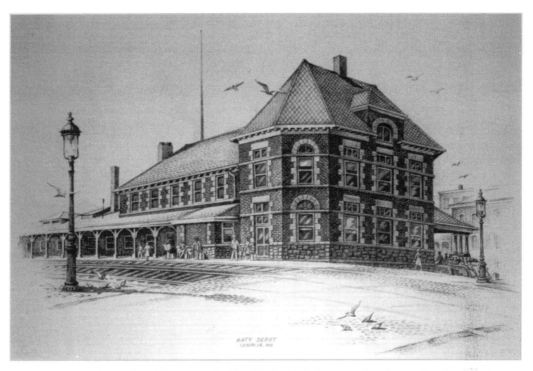

FIGURE 1.8 MKT Railroad Station in Sedalia 1895. This building replaced an earlier depot that was destroyed by fire.

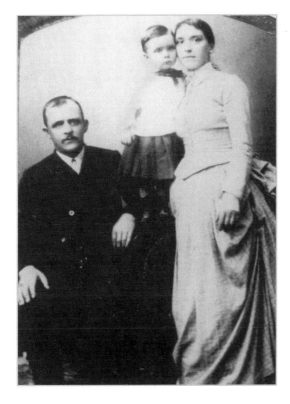

FIGURE 1.9 The young Dandy family in 1888.

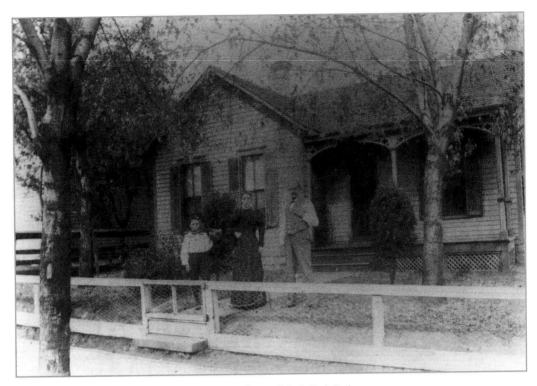

FIGURE 1.10   The Dandy Family in 1892 in front of their Sedalia home.

The family portrait (Figure 1.10) shows young Walter with his prized Bantam rooster in front of the family home. The family raised chickens in their yard. The house, which John referred to as "The Old Place." was located at 1325 East 5th Street, a block and a half east of Engineer Street, "so named because of the many railroad people in the vicinity. . . . It was a typical American railroad community with immigrants from England, Ireland, and Germany and other countries . . . "[11]

GRADE SCHOOL YEARS

In 1911, many years after this photograph (Figure 1.11) was taken, Walter's adoring mother, Rachel, wrote to him from England: "Pa has a little picture in his locket, one you had taken with your cap on when you were about eight years old. I heard him tell someone that was the brightest boy in the world."[12]

An account in the *Sedalia Democrat* describes young Walter playing "with boys in the neighborhood, including Stanley Battersby, making and flying kites, playing ball, swimming in the creek that was quite a distance away and to which they always walked. An expert marble player, which was a favorite game, he played for keeps and usually had a quart jar full of agates worth five and ten cents apiece by the time summer was over, which was quite an accumulation of wealth for a school boy."[13]

The account continues: "There were hairbreadth escapes, too, for young Dandy. Once he fell through the ice while ice skating, and, another time, when he was crawling

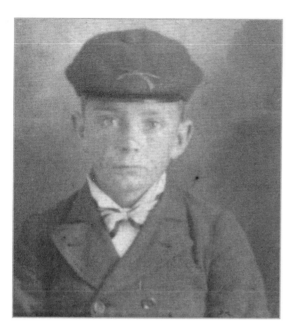

FIGURE 1.11   Walter as a schoolboy in 1892.

under a fence with his rabbit gun, it went off and the bullet whizzed by his ear, just barely missing it."

Walter was a good student and was allowed to skip a grade. He was small for his age, and a target for the larger boys, but legend has it that he could handle his own in a fight. The local boys, Walter among them, would occasionally watch a 10-cent show from the balcony of the old Woods Opera House.

The photograph (Figure 1.12) shows Walter in his schoolroom surrounded by class-mates who were from English, Irish, and German immigrant families. He is in the second

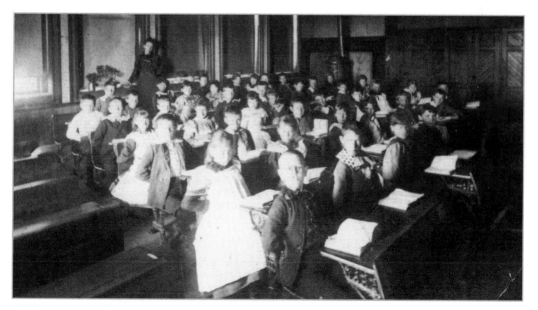

FIGURE 1.12   Walter in his classroom in the Summit School in Sedalia in 1892.

row on the far right. A family legend tells of the little boy who was so strong (and perhaps headstrong) that when he jiggled his foot in his schoolroom, the whole schoolhouse shook.

HIGH SCHOOL

According to records (or legends) at the *Sedalia Democrat,* Walter excelled as a newspaper carrier. "While he was attending high school, Walter Dandy was a carrier boy for the *Sedalia Democrat*—and, he didn't want to be just a carrier boy—he wanted to be the best carrier boy the paper had. He proved that he was, too, by winning consistently the Newsboy of the Month award during those years. He saved his money and invested in a bicycle, possibly pioneering the idea in Sedalia of delivery of paper by bicycle. This permitted him to have a much longer route and make more money."[14]

Years later (July 20, 1928), after passing through Sedalia on the train, he reflected[15]:

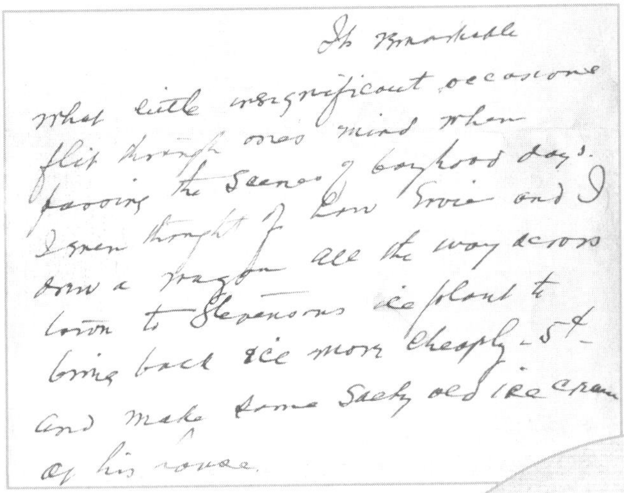

What little insignificant occasions
flit through ones mind when
passing the scenes of boyhood days.
I even thought of Low Grove and I
drove a wagon all the way across
town to Stevensons ice plant to
bring back ice more cheaply - 5¢ -
and make some Sachs old ice cream
of his course.

Walter graduated from Sedalia High School as valedictorian of his class in 1903. He gave a speech on "Education" at the ceremony in the Woods Opera House (Figures 1.13–1.15). His biographer William Lloyd Fox remarks: "At the time of his graduation he was of medium height, about 5 feet 8 inches and of a slight build." He also recounts that observers took note of the young man's "deep, penetrating blue eyes."[16]

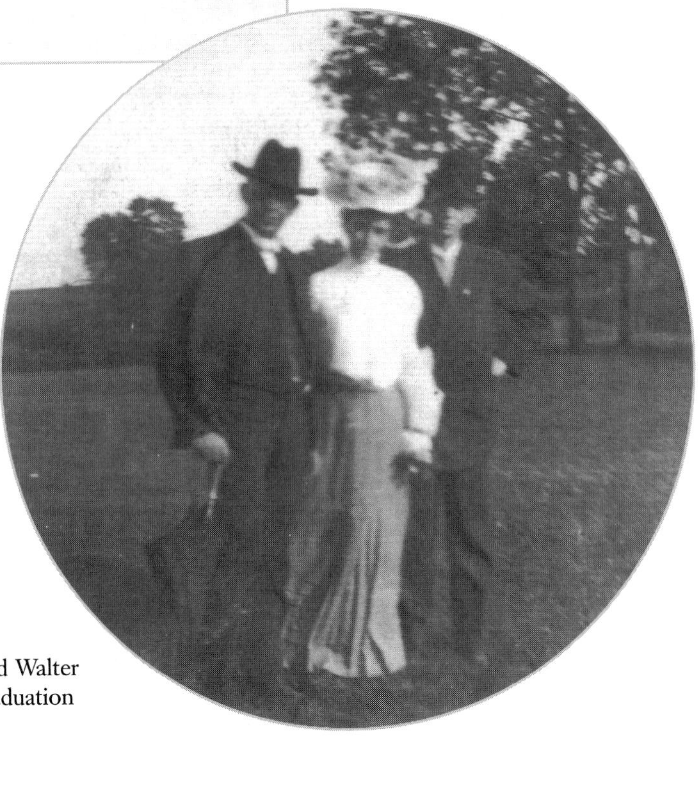

FIGURE 1.13 John, Rachel, and Walter Dandy at the time of Walter's graduation from high school in 1903.

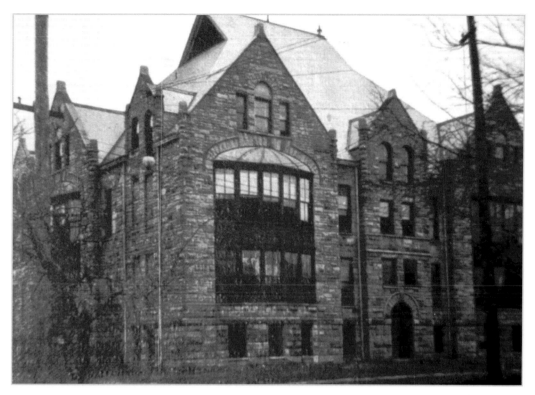

FIGURE 1.14   Sedalia High School.

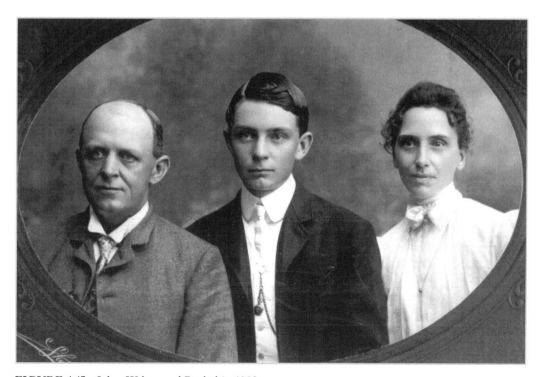

FIGURE 1.15   John, Walter, and Rachel in 1903.

UNIVERSITY OF MISSOURI

In September 1903, Walter entered the University of Missouri (Figure 1.16). In the upper part of the photograph, its well-known columns and adjacent quadrangle are visible. The columns are all that remain of the Academic Hall, the University's first and main building, which burned in 1892. The medical complex, which was completed in 1903, is in the lower right corner of the photograph. The University of Missouri was established in 1839 and was the first State university west of the Mississippi River. The Medical School was founded in 1872.[17]

Columbia, Missouri, at the time Walter Dandy entered college, was a small town (Figures 1.17–1.18). It is located 70 miles from Sedalia, just north of the Missouri River.

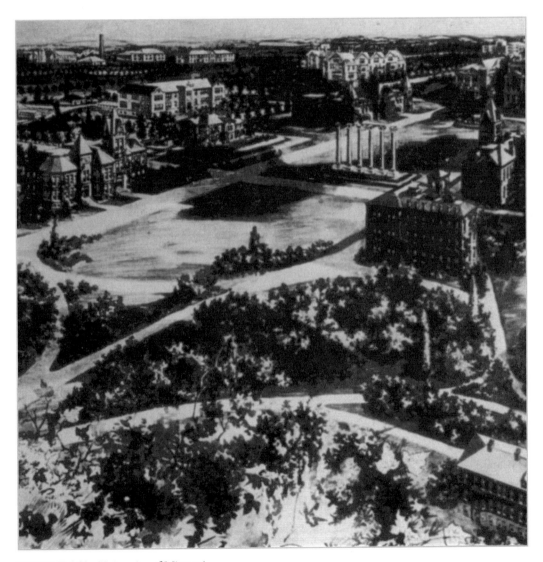

FIGURE 1.16   University of Missouri.

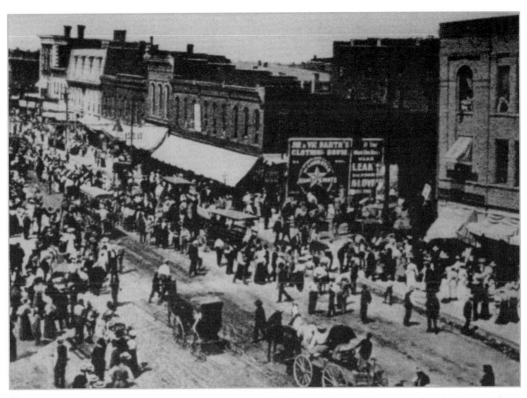

FIGURE 1.17   Columbia Missouri in the early 1900s. Scene of the county fair.

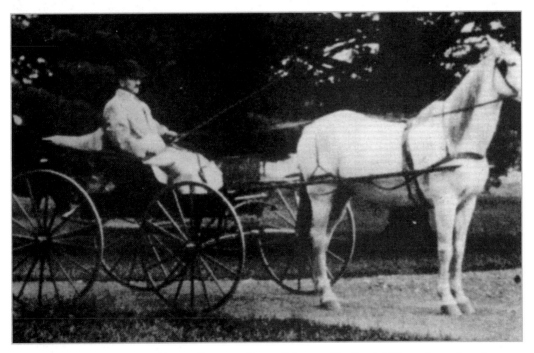

FIGURE 1.18   Walter probably saw "horse and buggy" doctors like Frank Nifong, shown here in Columbia in 1905.

LETTER FROM COLLEGE

Shortly after beginning classes at the University of Missouri, Walter wrote:[18]

September 10, 1903

Dear Mother and Father,

I have now passed three days at school. The time has been spent making entrance to the University which keeps you busy and running from one place to another waiting for the crowds for your turn.

The University is a grand set of buildings, about 12 in all, made of finest brick surrounded by pretty lawns and flowers and paved walks. There is a new building built for the medical students, and is equipped with every convenience.

There is a great crowd here but they all seem to be nice boys. It keeps you busy making acquaintances. We have also been very busy today putting down our carpet and fixing up our room which is now very nice. I believe the nicest in the club. The boarding club will not be open until Saturday. We have been boarding at a hotel downtown for $3.50 per week and get fine meals, except they don't give enough to fill my appetite. I don't think that is very high compared with prices here. You cannot get meals anyplace for less than 25¢ but we bought a ticket and got a reduction.

We were very lucky in getting our room. The persons who were in it before left several things (including much dirt), a fine brass bed, (the other beds are plain iron), a bureau and washstand, so we are pretty well fixed. I saved $5 by being valedictorian which, though small, nevertheless it helps out. I have about $27 left but have not bought any books yet. They are very high ranging from $10 to $15 but by joining a co-operative club you get them 10% or 1/10 cheaper. It costs $1 to join the club but you soon make more than that back.

I am getting the Democrat and Capital here by mail all right.

I have met many of the Sedalia boys and girls here.

Tomorrow our regular work begins. School runs from 8:30 A.M. to 4:30 P.M. I shall take English, German, Greek, Chemistry and Physics which keeps me as every one else is very busy all the time.

When did Papa go to work? Are you worrying? How is Mr. Battersby getting along? Joe Ikenberry is anxious for Stanley to come and keep him company. I think I will now close and go to bed. I am well and hope you are the same.

Your loving son, Walter E. Dandy

Do not expect too much from me in the letter line for you know I can not write a good letter. Write soon with lots of news.

Address U.B. Club, Columbia, MO

Friends at University of Missouri

Stanley Battersby described his roomate, Walter, during college years (Figures 1.19-1.21). Stanley recalled, "My hardest job as a roommate was to get him up for breakfast."[19] Stanley described "Walter's ability to organize his time, his intense concentration and his aggressiveness. After dinner on a typical day he would play cards until 7:30 in the evening, study intently until 10:00, then retire and immediately go to sleep—the latter two, in the presence of noisy social activity in his room. He allotted time for recreation, almost as faithfully as he did for work, a practice he continued through his entire life."[20]

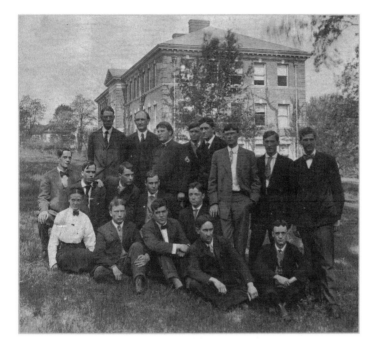

FIGURE 1.19 Walter and other students in front of Benton Hall. Walter is the third from the left in the middle row.

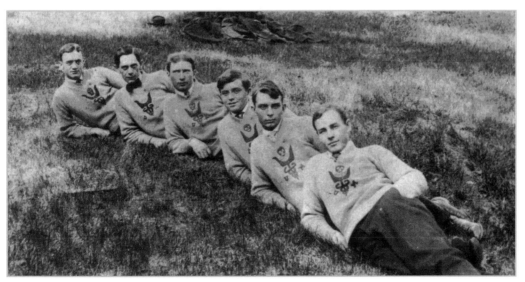

FIGURE 1.20 Walter and student friends. Walter is the second from the right.

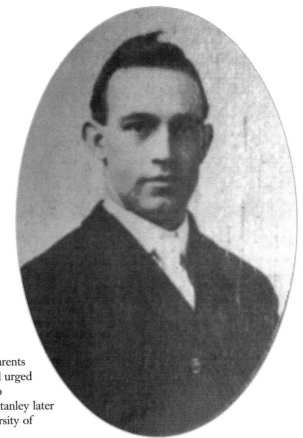

FIGURE 1.21 Stanley Battersby, Walter's college roommate from Sedalia. Stanley's parents were friends of John Dandy's in Barrow and urged John to move to Sedalia. Stanley went on to Hopkins Medical School in Walter's class. Stanley later became Professor of Pediatrics at the University of Missouri Medical School.

Eustice Semmes, MD, one of Walter's friends who later attended Johns Hopkins Medical School with him, remembers the college days: "We had the kind of relationship that promoted practical jokes that we played on each other, particularly during our first year there."[21] Years later, Dandy told his children about how the students brought a cow into the dormitory.

In the summers during college, Walter returned to Sedalia and worked jobs as a streetcar conductor, barn painter, and a nurse for a neighbor whom he referred to as "old man Larry."[22]

STUDENTS IN THE COUNTRY

During the college years, Walter enjoyed outings in the countryside, near Columbia Missouri. (Figures 1.22–1.24). He also learned to box, play baseball, golf, and the card game whist.

He learned the song "Hail Missouri," One of the two songs that made up his musical repertoire. (The other was "My Bonnie Lies Over the Ocean.") Fortunately for Walter Dandy's reputation, his performances of those songs were heard only by family members!

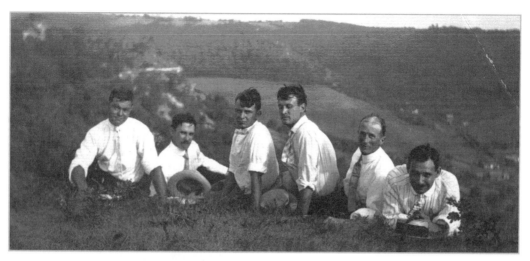

FIGURE 1.22   Walter is third from the left.

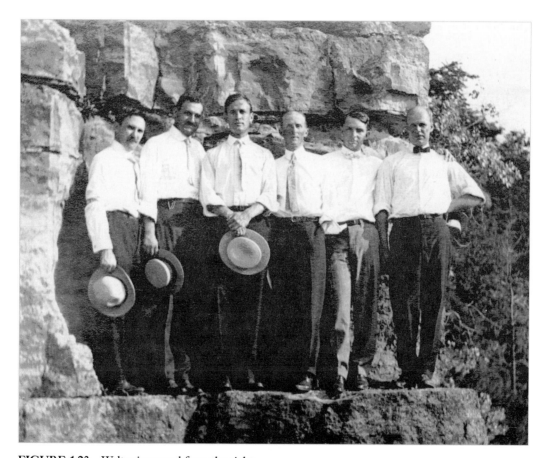

FIGURE 1.23   Walter is second from the right.

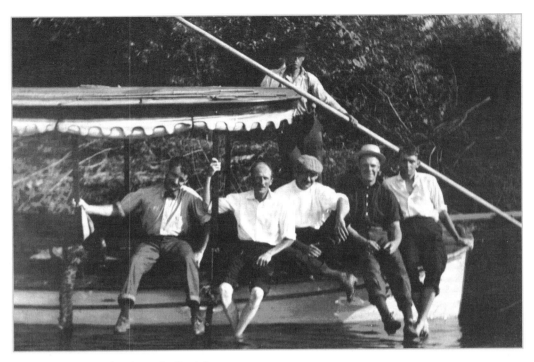

FIGURE 1.24   Walter is on the far right.

ACADEMIC LIFE AT UNIVERSITY OF MISSOURI

Walter was a very serious college student. His roommate, Stanley Battersby, commented that "he was constantly amazed at Walter's ability to concentrate."[23] Walter found it necessary to earn most of his expenses at the university. This proved to be a blessing in disguise because he was placed in laboratory jobs (Figure 1.25) that not only gave him an opportunity for scientific investigation, but also brought him into contact with Winterton C. Curtis, Professor of Zoology, who recognized Dandy's talents and encouraged him.

Another influential teacher was Professor George Lefevre (Figure 1.26). Like Curtis, he had earned his PhD at Johns Hopkins University. Dr LeFevre was Chairman of the Department of Zoology at the University of Missouri. Dandy always thought these two men were primarily responsible for his going to Hopkins. Walter applied for a Rhodes Scholarship. He succeeded in the initial selection, but because the University of Missouri had received the previous appointment for that region, did not receive the final appointment. Battersby said Dandy "took it in stride and I never heard him express any disappointment."[24] Both of his parents were disappointed at this for, despite the many faults they found with England, they wanted their son to have an English university education and even to live there.

In the meantime, Walter had written William Osler, Regius Professor of Medicine at Oxford who had left Hopkins two years before, to ask about the prospects of studying medicine at Oxford. Osler replied: "Dear Sir: To take the Oxford degree, you will first have to take the Oxford B.A. which would scarcely be worthwhile to spend that extra time. It would be very much better to finish at Johns Hopkins, and then come abroad for postgraduate work."[25] Walter took courses in the medical school during his junior and senior years and graduated with a total of 138 hours, 12 more than required. During his senior year, Walter applied to Johns Hopkins Medical School and was accepted as a second year student because of his advanced courses at the University of Missouri.

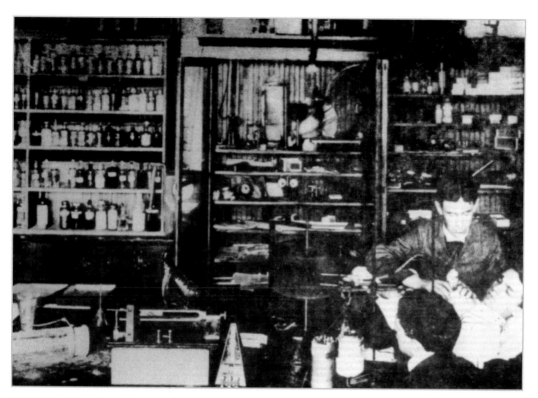

FIGURE 1.25   Physiology Lab at the University of Missouri in 1897.

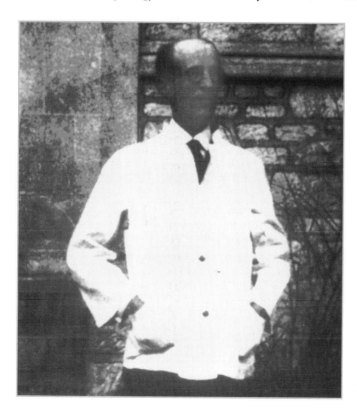

FIGURE 1.26   George LeFevre, Ph.D., Professor of Zoology, Chairman of the Department of Zoology, University of Missouri. Lefevre had an important effect on Walter's career.

GRADUATION

Walter graduated from the University of Missouri in 1907 (Figure 1.27). His honors included election to Phi Beta Kappa and Sigma Xi, an honorary scientific society. He was also named as one of the "First Five," and QEBH, a society of the University of Missouri limited to ten people. In addition, he served as President of the Pettis County Club, a social club (Figure 1.28).

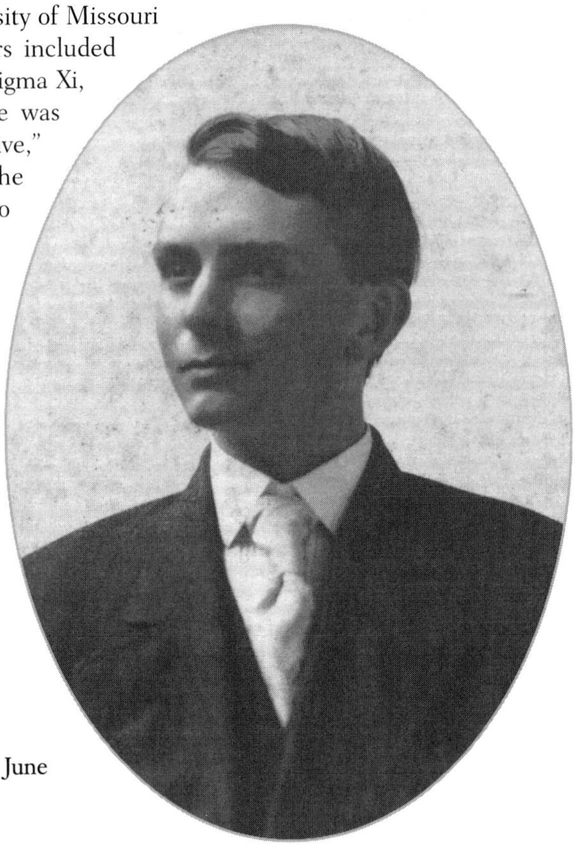

FIGURE 1.27 Walter E. Dandy upon his graduation from the University of Missouri, in June 1907, Sigma Xi.

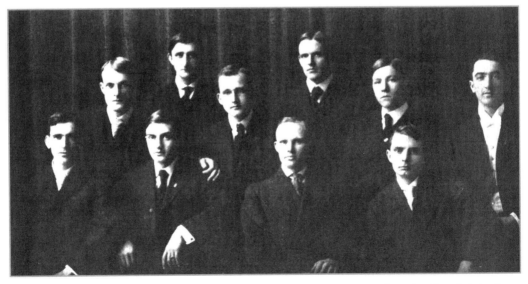

FIGURE 1.28 Pettis County Club at the University of Missouri (1907–1908). Walter Dandy is in the front row, far right.

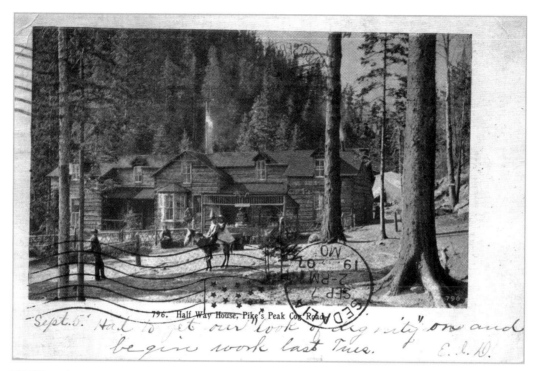

FIGURE 1.29   Half Way House, Pike's Peak, Colorado: postcard sent in 1907 to Sedalia.

TRIP FOLLOWING COLLEGE GRADUATION

Before entering medical school, Walter took a train trip from Sedalia through Denver where he saw Pike's Peak (Figure 1.29), the Garden of the Gods, and Cripple Creek. Near Denver, he marveled at the famous "Georgetown Loop . . . the most beautiful and awe-inspiring trip I ever took, It was my first view of mountains from near at hand." He also went to San Francisco, Los Angeles, Salt Lake City, and Seattle. Later, he noted, ". . . the blocks in Salt Lake City are 2 1/2 Sedalia blocks long or 7 blocks to the mile."[26]

He arrived in Baltimore to attend Johns Hopkins School of Medicine in September 1907.

℮DITORIAL ℭOMMENT

A Personal Letter To Walter E. Dandy
By John J. Oro, M.D.

Dear Walter,

Excuse me for using the familiar, but as I strive to know you, it seems to me that you would not mind. The letters, words, and pictures in this book, lovingly organized by your family and admirers, further illuminate your story. This is what I have come to learn about your life in Missouri.

Your years in Missouri reveal that you were energetic, intelligent, and enjoyed the full richness of life: family, friends, games, craft and work, the occasional prank, curiosity, and creativity. The pioneering spirit you showed in your neurosurgical career was probably related to your own father's closeness to adventure. Economic hard times in northern England during the 1880s caused your father and mother, John & Rachel Dandy, to consider moving across an ocean, the question was, which one? As a railroad man, there were opportunities for your father in Australia and Africa, but due to the encouragement of his friend and fellow railroad man Robert Battersby, who had previously moved to Sedalia, Missouri, John, and later Rachel, emigrated to America.

They settled in Sedalia, a bustling railroad and manufacturing town in western Missouri. Sedalia had been established in 1860, just 23 years prior to your father's arrival, by General George R. Smith who had named it for his daughter "Sed," born Sarah.[1] In 1882, one year prior to your father's arrival, Sedalia was a "a city so well-known abroad and at home, so well established in character, growing so surely and swiftly, having now all the conditions and concomitants which guarantee that she will be a city of 30,000 people within the next ten years...."[2] Here, your father found work as a fireman on the Missouri, Kansas & Texas Railroad, a line whose early history is filled with a "wealth of romance and adventure."[3] He later worked as an engineer on its renowned passenger train, the Katy Flyer, the "Fast Train to Indian Territory, Texas, Mexico and Pacific Coast Resorts."[4]

It was in this setting that you were born on April 6, 1886. Your biographer, William Lloyd Fox, describes you as "bright, active boy" and "one of the best students at Summit School."[5] Your love of sports and competition were apparent early: marbles, tennis, ice-skating, swimming, and baseball. Your industry must have been noticed by your community as you delivered the St. Louis paper in the morning and two routes of the Sedalia Democrat in the evening, excelling at the task by using the latest technology, the bicycle![6] (Even the title of the article by Dr. Robert L. Glass of Sedalia, published in December 1965 in Missouri Medicine—"Walter Dandy, Sedalia's Number One Paperboy"—recalls your prowess.[7])

Apparently, you also excelled in carpentry. R. Stanley "Bat" Battersby, your lifelong friend, "clearly remembers a small wooden bench Walter made as a boy, a bench so precisely mortised and flawlessly finished that it could have passed for the work of a journeyman cabinet maker."[8] After graduating from high school as valedictorian in 1903, you moved to Columbia to attend the University of Missouri. With a population of 5,600, Columbia was known as an educational center with six schools: the state university, two women's colleges, a bible college, as well as two academies.

Thirteen years before you arrived, the University had been seriously challenged. Its main building, known as Academic Hall, had been built in 1880. As the Athenian Society was gathering in the chapel on the evening of January 9, 1892, a short circuit in the ceiling started a fire that caused the central chandelier to come crashing down.[9] No one was injured. Fortunately, the university was in the hands of the indomitable Richard Henry Jesse, who just five months earlier had been appointed as the seventh, and youngest, president of the university. His announcement: "The main building of the University of the State of Missouri was totally destroyed by fire on Saturday evening, 9 January, but the University itself—its learning, its skill, its zeal, its enthusiasm—remains untouched, and its work will go on without interruption."[10] Classes resumed without delay in buildings all around Columbia. Jesse rebuilt the university and, by the time you arrived, as written in your first letter home, you found a "grand set of buildings, about 12 in all, made of the finest brick...."[11] Laid out in a quadrangle, the buildings bordered an expanse of lawn; at its center stood the 6 great Ionic columns of Academic Hall. They are now emblematic of the university itself.

Continued

EDITORIAL COMMENT *Continued*

Your roommate in Benton Hall was none other than your Sedalia friend "Bat" Battersby, son of your family friends Robert Battersby and his wife who had influenced your parents move to America. In addition to your studies, you continued to play baseball, took up golf, and even tried boxing. Summers brought you back to Sedalia to work as a barn painter and a conductor on a trolley line. Older residents later remember you as "the best conductor in town and the best painter of the biggest barns."[12]

As a junior, you enrolled in The Medical Department of the University of Missouri, which, in 1872, had been reorganized and moved to the Columbia campus. Andrew W. McAlester, professor of surgery and materia medica, had become dean in 1880 and expanded the school to a three-year program in 1890, and a four-year program in 1898.[13] For his central role in establishing and expanding the school, we now recognized him as "the father of the University of Missouri School of Medicine."[14]

The "New Medical Building", that we now know as McAlester Hall, had been completed in 1903, two years prior to your arrival on campus. It housed the medical library, offices, aquaria, animal rooms, mechanical shop, lecture and research rooms, and laboratories for the basic science departments. It was here that you spent two years studying medicine. The picture of you and your fellow students on the lawn in front of the McAlester building (page—), speaks volumes to us. You compiled an excellent record and developed close ties to you mentors, professors of zoology George Lefevre and Winterton C. Curtis. However, being a serious student did not keep you from pulling a prank or two. Remember when Dean McAlester asked you, then president of Benton Hall, about a cow that was brought into the hall? He told you to take care of the problem. You said you would; of course, as Sadie later told me, you had brought the cow in yourself.[15]

Toward the end of your second year in medical school, you wrote to Sir William Osler about studying medicine at Oxford. Osler recommended you train at Johns Hopkins. With the support of your mentors Lefevre, Curtis, and Dr. W. J. Calvert, all graduates of Johns Hopkins, you were accepted into the second year class.[16] You graduated from MU on June 5, 1907, second in your class of over 100 and moved to Baltimore to begin your studies. It must have been fun to have two of your classmates move with you: Thomas Grover Orr and Raphael Eustace Semmes, destined to become the first neurosurgeon to practice neurological surgery in Memphis.[17]

Even as you developed your legendary career at Johns Hopkins, you maintained very close ties with Missouri. Between the first and second year of your studies, you returned to Columbia to assist professors Lefevre and Curtis in their zoological research. You donated funds to help Professor Curtis send his students to summer research fellowships at the Marine Biological Laboratory at Woods Hole, Massachusetts. Your personal qualities and talents were increasingly recognized as evidenced by your service on the Medical School Foundation board of trustees and on the Advisory Council for the Board of Curators.

In 1928, at the age of 42, you were awarded the Honorary Degree of Doctor of Laws for your contributions to the University. It must have been a wonderful occasion. As you noted: "that this honor should first come from my Alma Mater will always be a source of great pride and satisfaction."[18] Since you left us in 1946, we continue to remember. Articles have been written about you and a biography has detailed your life. At University of Missouri Health Sciences Center in Columbia we named the new neurosurgical intensive care unit in your honor. One morning I was sitting having breakfast at the hospital cafeteria with a colleague of mine, Dr. Jerry Templer. As I explained the plans for our new neurosurgical unit, he suggested that we name it after you. Jerry, an otolaryngologist with a weekly clinic in Sedalia, knew you where born there and had even driven past the house in which you grew up. The suggestion was so obvious, that I was chagrined I had not thought of it myself. The gears started spinning and in a few months we had the approval from the Chancellor of the Columbia campus and University President.

The Walter E. Dandy Neurosurgical Intensive Care Unit was inaugurated on January 23, 1986, 100 years after your birth. Your lovely wife, Sadie, and your physician son, Dr. Walter Dandy, Jr., were present at the conference and reception as were friends or admirers including Drs. Edward R Laws, Jr., Donlin M. Long, Hugo V. Rizzoli, and Hugh E. Stephenson.[19] A precious moment occurred at the end of the conference when Sadie came to the front of the auditorium carrying a brown paper bag.

Continued

She stated to Dr. Clark Watts, then chief of neurosurgery, that she had something to give to the Division, but that she had not had time to wrap it. All were puzzled over what the bag contained. The audience fell silent when she pulled out the honorary hood that had been given to you by the University of Missouri 58 years earlier.

In these pages you will find some places, diversions, adventures, honors, and accomplishments of your life. They are essential to us as we come to know you better. Certainly, friends and mentors, exemplified by your lifelong friendships with Stanley Battersby and your professors George Lefevre and Winterton C. Curtis, played a central role. But, through these words and images, we sense that your "greatest source of pleasure was a close and happy family."[20]

Sincerely,

John J. Oro

February 2002

CHAPTER 2

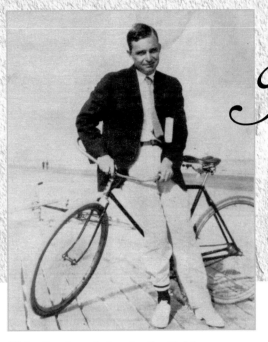

The Making of a Surgeon 1907–1922

Walter Dandy on the boardwalk with bike.

CHAPTER 2 OUTLINE

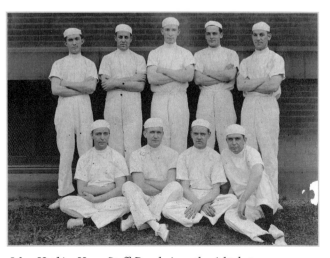

Johns Hopkins House Staff. Dandy is on the right, bottom row.

THE JOHNS HOPKINS HOSPITAL

When Walter Dandy arrived at Johns Hopkins in 1907, the hospital had been in operation for only eighteen years, the medical school for only fourteen years. For the next thirty-nine years, the medical school and the hospital were to be the center of his life. He studied there, carried on research, performed surgery, saw patients, and even lived under the rotunda during his internship and residency. A hospital elevator, says family tradition, was the scene of his first meeting with his future wife, and their four children were born in the Maternity Area of the Hopkins Women's Clinic. At the time of his death in 1946, his son Walter was a second-year student at the medical school.

A short history of the hospital is an integral part of Dr. Dandy's personal, as well as professional, history.

Johns Hopkins, the chief benefactor of the hospital and the university, was born in southern Maryland in 1795. Moving from the wholesale grocery business to banking and railroad enterprises, he amassed a fortune. A Quaker and a philanthropist, Hopkins wanted to build a hospital to help the poor. He bought thirteen acres in East Baltimore on what was then called Loudenschlager's Hill. The site had been a mental hospital (then called an insane asylum) before the patients were moved to a location near Catonsville. He designated $7 million in his will to be divided equally between the hospital and the university that would bear his name.

When Hopkins died in 1873, the old hospital had been razed and the site prepared for building, but he was never to see even a blueprint for his new hospital. The Queen Anne style building was designed by John Shaw Billings, a Georgetown physician and hospital and public health expert (Figure 2.1). The building was started in 1877 and finished twelve years later. The hospital opened in 1889 and was the first in the country to have central heating.

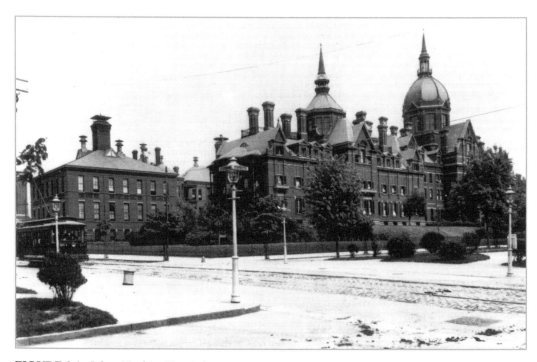

FIGURE 2.1   Johns Hopkins Hospital.

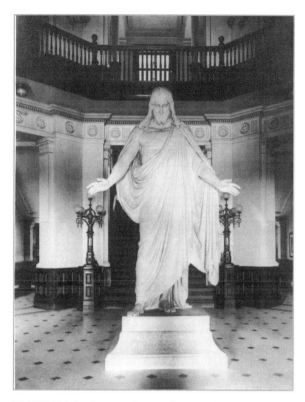

FIGURE 2.2   Statue of Jesus Christ in the Rotunda of the Johns Hopkins Hospital copy of statue by Bertel Thorwaldsen, 1821. The inscription reads: "Come Unto Me all ye that are weary and heavy laden and I will give you rest."

Cleanliness was an important feature of its design. To ensure sanitary maintenance, every inside corner was to be rounded to avoid the buildup of dust, dirt, and dead insects in crevices. Although the term "germ" was used at that time, most people were not sure what it meant. It was still widely believed that illnesses were caused by miasma—poisonous vapors that rose from the soil. The heating and ventilating systems were designed to purify the air. No elevators were built initially because of the danger of the vapors.

Fortunately, though, for the existence of the Dandy children, elevators had been installed by 1923. When the children were young, they often visited the hospital, sometimes to visit patients, sometimes to watch their father operate, and sometimes to have their own wounds and illnesses treated. They may not have understood the scope of the hospital's mission, but two of its messages were clear. The inscription on the sundial outside the entrance reads, "One hour alone is in thy hands; the hour on which the shadow stands." The other message, is the outstretched, welcoming arms of the statue of Christ just inside the hospital entrance (Figure 2.2).

The sculpture of Christ is a 10-foot copy of Thorwaldsen's original in Copenhagen. Made of Carrara marble, it speaks the promise of compassion and release from suffering to all who enter. Some believed that the statue "was sought to offset criticism from the more conservative element in late nineteenth century Baltimore that the hospital had no religious affiliation."[1] In recent years, members of the Dandy family visiting the hospital saw Post-it Notes attached to the statue's feet, apparently from patients seeking help.

JOHNS HOPKINS UNIVERSITY MEDICAL SCHOOL

The Medical School was opened four years after the hospital, its construction delayed by an economic depression. It owed its buildings, in large part, to the feminist movement; it owed its unique qualities of instruction to the four physicians shown in the John Singer Sargent group portrait (Figure 2.3).

Long before the medical school was built, Hopkins' first president, Daniel Gilman, and the Johns Hopkins trustees wanted to emphasize innovations. In the United States at that time, future doctors were taught by part-time practicing local physicians. The trustees wanted a full-time medical faculty whose members were researchers as well as professors teaching in a four-year curriculum. The four doctors in the portrait were hired as professors between 1884 and 1889. All were between thirty-one and thirty-nine years of age at the time they were hired. Together and separately, the "Big Four" had a profound and lasting influence on American medical education.

To raise the funds needed to build the Medical School, the trustees sought assistance, and four wealthy Baltimore women came forward with an offer to help: Martha Carey Thomas, Mary Elizabeth Garrett, Elizabeth King, and Mary Gwinn. The women were daughters of the original trustees—unmarried, wealthy, well-educated, and devoted to the feminist movement (Figure 2.4). They would raise the $500,000 needed to open the school and pay for a medical school building if the following conditions were met: (1) the school must open its doors to qualified women; (2) all students must have a college degree; (3) competitive merit must determine student selection; and, (4) regular assessment of performance by examination must occur.[2] The trustees had no problem with the last three, but were unsure about the first condition. They had no choice but to accept the offer. Among the professors, all signed the agreement except Welch. By 1892, the money was in hand. The Johns Hopkins School of Medicine opened in 1893.

The Medical School curriculum emphasized the scientific method, bedside teaching and laboratory research, and joint medical school and hospital appointments. The new method also instituted standardized advanced training in specialized fields of medicine with the creation of the first house staff fellowships and postgraduate internships.

Mary Garrett commissioned John Singer Sargent to paint the portrait of the four doctors. The painting was done in London in 1905 because William Osler was at Oxford at that time. The other three came to London to sit for the painting at Sargent's studio.

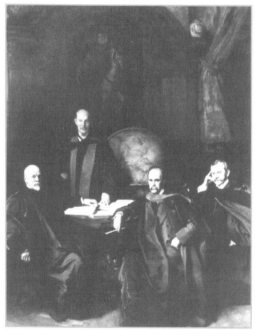

FIGURE 2.3 *The Four Doctors* painted by John Singer Sargent: Front row: Dr. William H. Welch (pathologist), Dr. William Osler (internist), Dr. Howard Kelly (gynecologist). Behind: Dr. William S. Halsted (surgeon).

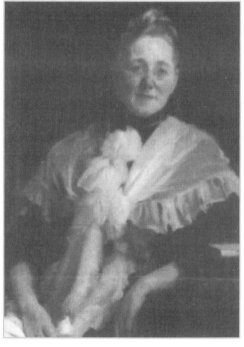

FIGURE 2.4 Mary Elizabeth Garrett and the Women's Fund Committee raised the money needed to open the Johns Hopkins School of Medicine.

DANDY ENTERS MEDICAL SCHOOL

The Medical School curriculum introduced by the Big Four, with its strong emphasis on experiential learning, was perfect for Walter Dandy's temperament. He was active and intensely focused, full of curiosity, and eager for the kind of challenges that the real world could offer. "Study was rigorous, including unprecedented hours of bedside learning at the side of experts, original research projects guided by respected clinicians, and extensive laboratory training."[3] He had second-year standing when he entered because of his work at the medical school in Missouri (Figures 2.5, 2.6, and 2.7). He was accompanied by two classmates from Missouri, Eustace Semmes and Thomas Orr.

Walter had begun writing to his parents when he first left home to go to the University of Missouri. It was a practice that he maintained with consistency until the end of their lives. The interchange provides us with valuable insights into his development as a doctor and as a person. For example, a letter from his mother suggests the change in Walter's state of mind, away from his confined, preoccupied existence in Missouri. "I just like these English people [Battersby and others] to know that you have come out of your snail box [a term she attributed to the Battersbys] and [are] now on a far way to be the leading man in the country. I really believe you will. You have the ability and the money to get the highest in your profession. It is a pleasure for us to give you anything you need."[4]

The letter shows how much emotional (and financial) support his mother offered her son, and shows as well her faith in him and her ambition for his future. In another letter, she also steered her son toward the value of certain personal qualities. She drew his attention to the importance of affection and attentiveness to others, evoking the writings of Osler (who, although gone from Hopkins had left an important legacy). "[He] seems

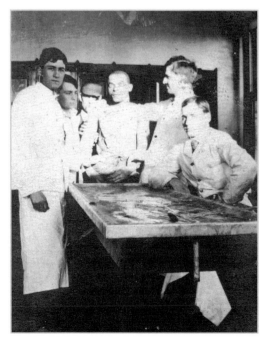 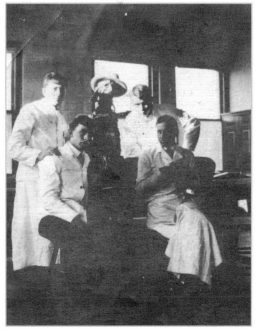

FIGURE 2.5 The School of Medicine Anatomy Lab. Dandy is second from the left.

FIGURE 2.6 The School of Medicine: Anatomy Lab. Dandy is on the upper right.

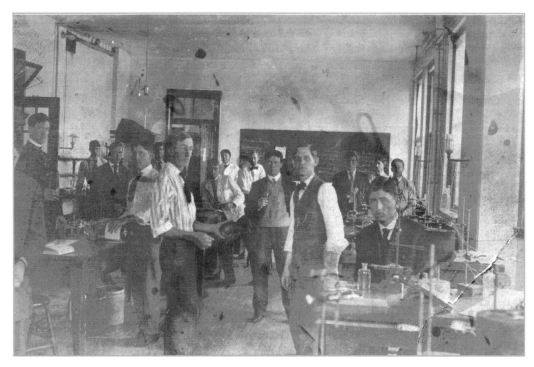

FIGURE 2.7   The Anatomy Lab. Dandy is at the center, leaning on table.

to be a very affectionate fatherly man that has the students' interests at heart. It says for students to keep their affections in cold storage. . . ."[5]

During the summer of 1908, Dandy worked with his former professors George Lefevre and W. C. Curtis on a research project on reproduction and artificial propagation of freshwater mussels. Their floating laboratory was the stern-wheeler *Curlew*, on the Mississippi river near La Crosse, Wisconsin. During this summer, according to his biographer Fox, in his leisure time, Dandy learned to play poker.[6]

THE "DANDY EMBRYO"

By the end of his first trimester at Hopkins, Dandy had attracted the attention of his anatomy professor, Dr. Franklin P. Mall. Mall (Figure 2.8), a Leipzig-trained anatomist, had been

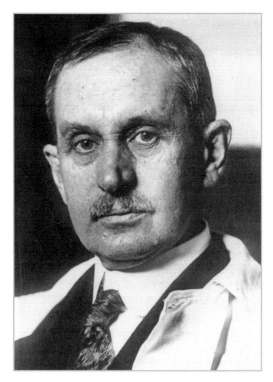

FIGURE 2.8   Franklin P. Mall, Professor of Anatomy, Johns Hopkins Medical School.

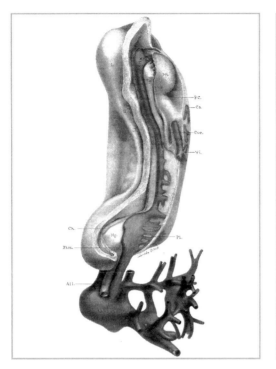

FIGURE 2.9   *Dandy Embryo*: drawing by Dorothy Peters, who had studied with Max Broedel.

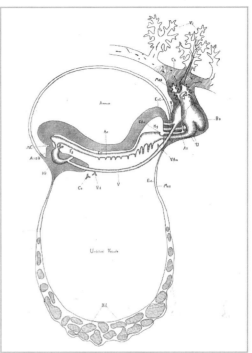

FIGURE 2.10   *Dandy Embryo* showing the yolk sac, drawing by Walter Dandy.

hired by Dr. Welch to become Professor of Anatomy at Hopkins. He became one of the leading anatomists of his day.

Noticing Dandy's interest in the field (Dandy had considered becoming an anatomist during college) and his talent for drawing, Mall asked his student to reconstruct and describe an embryo of twenty-one days, one of the youngest human embryos in his collection. The work led to Dandy's first article, published in 1911. (See Appendix D)

The article was illustrated by a colored drawing (Figure 2.9) by Dorothy Peters, and by Dandy's black-and-white drawings of the embryo (Figure 2.10). The work was important to Dandy, as is evident from the many comments in correspondence to his parents. Hopkins recognized the importance of his publication by awarding him a Master's degree in 1910, five months before his graduation from medical school. Subsequent medical literature contains references to the "Dandy Embryo."

Medical School: Work at the Hunterian

As a student, Dandy spent much of his time at the Hunterian Laboratory of Experimental Medicine (Figure 2.11 and 2.12). This laboratory was to have been named for Françoiso Magendie, a French physiologist associated with animal surgery, but strong opposition from antivivisectionists in Baltimore led the authorities to name it instead for John Hunter, a famous English surgeon. (The antivivisectionists were undeterred; they continued to haunt and taunt Hopkins medical researchers during the first decades of the twentieth century.)

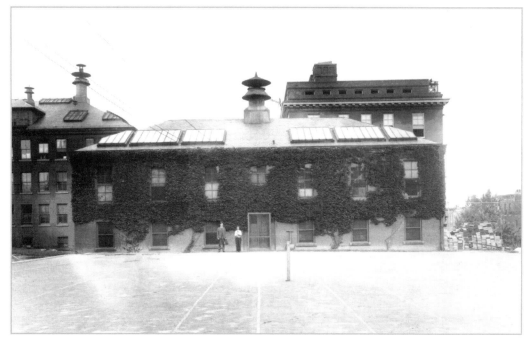

FIGURE 2.11   The Hunterian Laboratory of Experimental Medicine.

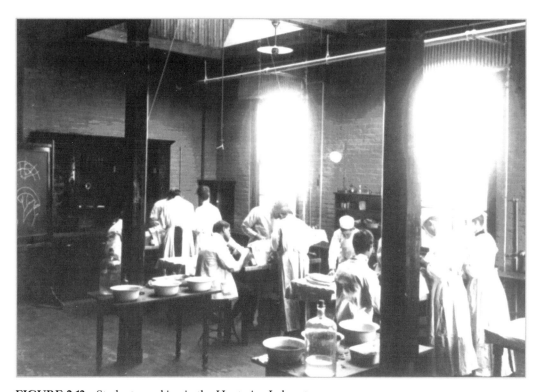

FIGURE 2.12   Students working in the Hunterian Laboratory.

As Halsted's assistant resident in 1896, Harvey Cushing had been instrumental in the establishment of the Hunterian Laboratory and supervised it until he left Hopkins in 1912. As a medical student, Dandy's ability in anatomy and surgery had drawn Cushing's attention. Dandy sought, and apparently obtained, Cushing's consent to do research in the laboratory during his senior year of medical school for the work on the "Dandy Embryo."

Dandy graduated from medical school in 1910, standing seventeenth in a class of eighty-five.[7] His connection with Cushing, however, was not over.

The Young Doctor's First Year

After graduating from medical school, Dandy went to Sedalia to visit his parents (Figure 2.13). Dandy's mother wrote that she felt he needed to "loaf to recuperate after the trying ordeal of the exams. You are young and can't stand it like Dr. Cushing, a man of mature years."[8] (Cushing was seventeen years older than Dandy.) But his vacation was cut short because Cushing wanted him to begin work as an assistant in surgery in the Hunterian.

At the Hunterian, Cushing assigned Dandy and Emile Goetsch research on the origins and distribution of the blood vessels and the nerves to the pituitary gland of the dog. Their findings were published as "The Blood Supply of the Pituitary Body," in the *American Journal of Anatomy*, in 1910–1911. (See Appendix A)[9] This was Dandy's second article of the 160 published during his lifetime. Dandy himself did "the beautiful drawings in the papers [Figure 2.14] with coaching from Max Broedel."[10]

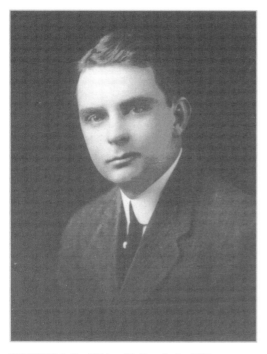

FIGURE 2.13   Walter E. Dandy in 1909.

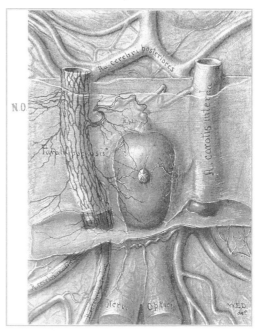

FIGURE 2.14   *Nerve supply of the Pituitary*, drawing by Dandy, 1913.

During this time, John and Rachel discussed leaving Sedalia and moving to Baltimore. In October 1910, Rachel, who seemed to have had no difficulty with the decision, wrote: "Well we have decided to come to Baltimore. I am getting anxious for Pa to quit. I feel he has worked long enough and it is not necessary for him to work for the purpose of accumulating wealth."[11] John retired at 54. At the time, he seemed ready enough to overcome his misgivings: "I have decided to quit running an engine for a living. Having decided to make the interest on money keep me. Myself and wife are staying in Baltimore with our son who is a Doctor in Johns Hopkins University. We have been here about 2 months. At the first I thought I could not be satisfied unless I was on an engine, but now I find it is no trouble."[12] But his later writings revealed a real ambivalence about the move, admitting that he was "not well satisfied. Nothing to do and [had] led a busy life."[13] He confessed to a friend living in Portland, Oregon, "I almost feel I would like it better there [Portland] than here [Baltimore]." Their son found John and Rachel a house to rent in Baltimore, where they stayed for almost a year before setting sail in October 1911 to visit their families in England and Ireland.

Halsted's Staff

Young Dr. Dandy served on Halsted's staff at the Hunterian from 1910 until 1912. The first year of Dandy's service as resident "sharpened rather than dulled Dr. Dandy's interest in investigative work. Dr. Halsted recognized his unusual gifts and encouraged and stimulated him."[14] Halsted influenced Dandy profoundly both as a surgeon and as a mentor.

Halsted was a shy man and an indifferent lecturer, but he was a brilliant clinician and surgeon. Dandy learned from him the importance of personal habits of fastidiousness. Dandy's requirements for polished shoes, clean fingernails, and care in clothing were enforced not only with those who worked for him, but with his children as well.

Following is a tribute to William Halsted, excerpted from Donlin M. Long.[15]

> William Halsted developed the field of surgery as we know it today. Even though anesthesia and antisepsis had allowed elective surgery to become a reality, the slash-and-burn technique of surgery practiced since ancient times was slow to disappear. Halsted changed all this with his emphasis upon meticulous hemostasis, anatomic dissection, and reconstruction with gentle tissue handling. The surgical techniques that are now the basis of all operative therapy did not exist before Halsted. . . . He created various specialty areas of surgery. . . . He allowed Cushing to develop neurosurgery, although he expressed his skepticism about the viability of this aspect of surgery. . . . Halsted and Osler conceived the concept of formal residency training, which Halsted put into practice.

Other sources tell a good story about another of Halsted's contributions—the use of rubber gloves. After his surgical nurse Caroline Hampton developed dermatitis from the cleaning solutions used in the operating room, Halsted asked the Goodyear Rubber Company to make two pairs of thin rubber gloves for her. The gloves were so successful that they were ordered for others. And, apparently Miss Hampton was so grateful that she consented to become Halsted's wife in 1890.

During Walter Dandy's first two years on Halsted's house staff, Harvey Cushing was the Chief Resident (Figure 2.15).

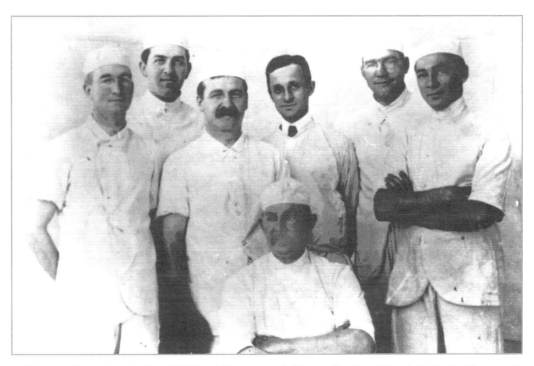

FIGURE 2.15   Halsted and staff: Halsted (front center), Harvey Cushing (directly behind without cap).

A Conflict Develops: A Researcher Establishes Himself

As in his medical school years, Dandy's immediate supervisor at the Hunterian in 1910–1911 was Harvey Cushing. In 1911–1912, Dandy became Cushing's clinical assistant working under Halsted. "Both Cushing and Dandy were high strung, temperamental individuals and their personalities clashed on many occasions during the year in the Hunterian Laboratory. The following year in the hospital was not a happy one for Dandy."[16]

In 1912, Cushing was planning to move to Boston to take a position at Harvard. He had made offers to several young men, including Dandy, to work with him in Boston. Shortly before Cushing left, however, he informed Dandy that he would not be taking Dandy to Boston after all. Cushing's change of mind left Dandy without a position for the following year. According to his colleague Samuel Crowe, "Just before Cushing left for Harvard, he told Dandy he was not going to take him along. Dr. Halsted had been told Dandy was going with Cushing so he had filled all the positions on his house staff."[17] Dr. Winfred Smith, director of the hospital, called Dandy into his office. Smith said that he would find room in the hospital, and that he would find out Dandy's status from Halsted.

Halsted rescued Dandy, finding him a place on his surgical staff (Figure 2.16). One of the reasons given was Dandy's impressive and original experiments on hydrocephalus. While living in the hospital, Dandy had begun work in the Hunterian with Kenneth Blackfan, a resident in pediatrics. Their task was to search for the origin, circulation, and absorption of cerebrospinal fluid and the cause of hydrocephalus. They were able to produce hydrocephalus in experimental animals by blocking the aqueduct of Sylvius.

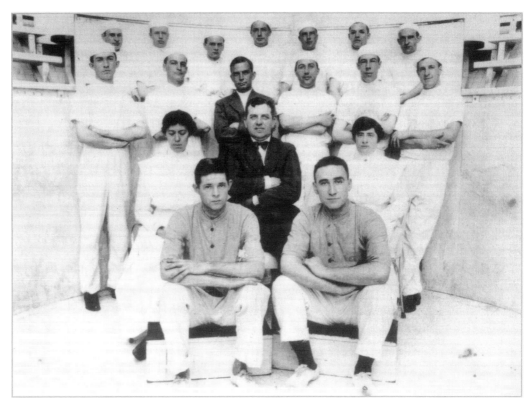

FIGURE 2.16   Johns Hopkins Hospital surgical house staff: Dandy is in second row from the top, center, wearing a dark jacket.

In 1913, three years after his graduation, Dandy reported his fundamental studies on hydrocephalus. The medical world acknowledged that his findings provided a break-through to understanding of the disorder. In 1914 Dandy and Blackfan published the results of their research. Chapter 4 discusses this work.

PERSPECTIVES ON THE CUSHING AND DANDY CONFLICT

Much (maybe too much) has been written about the Dandy–Cushing controversy, including an article written in 1994, "New Observations on the Dandy–Cushing Controversy" by Eugene S. Flamm, M.D.[18]

Figure 2.17 shows Cushing and Dandy at Jekyll Island, Georgia, before a tennis match. "Cushing had the form, but Dandy won the game," was the remark attributed to Mrs. Harry Slack, Jr. who took the photograph.[19]

According to Fox, the controversy began during the academic year 1910–1911, when Cushing challenged Dandy's research methods and disagreed about the findings on stim-ulation of the sympathetics.[20]

Numerous other flare-ups occurred in that year and the year following. When Dandy had written about them in a letter to his mother (who was in England), she counseled patience:

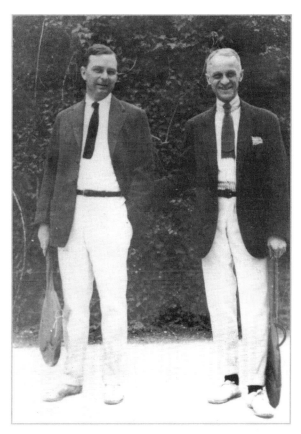

FIGURE 2.17 Dandy and Cushing at Jekyll Island in 1921.

"Very glad you are having such good work even though it is with a hard master. Never mind. Some day you will be your own master and can do just as you please. But in the meantime you must submit to the powers above you and Cushing that would spoil your future. His wonderful operations must be very trying on his quick irritable temper so you must overlook his temper. It is the great strain of his work that makes him so irritable. Probably you would be the same if in his position."[21]

Cushing and Dandy came from very different backgrounds. Cushing entered Yale in 1886 at the age of 17, the same year Walter Dandy was born. Cushing's great grandfather, grandfather, father, and brother were physicians. Dandy's immigrant parents were relatively uneducated. His father left school in the third grade and his mother finished high school. Dandy was the first in his family to attend college.

Their surgical styles were also different. Cushing was careful, precise, and methodical. Dandy was, according to neurosurgeon Edward Laws, "inspired and intuitive."[22] Describing their personal traits, Laws continued: "Both men were less than ideal in a variety of ways, but is this not the rule for geniuses, great statesmen, Nobel laureates, and individuals responsible for scientific revolutions? . . . Intolerance, stubbornness, competitiveness, and the inability to accept criticism probably were essential to other qualities that engendered the successes of Cushing. Similarly, impulsiveness, boldness, and individualism were all part and parcel of the brilliance Dandy displayed as an innovative neurosurgeon."[23]

In the long run, Cushing's rejection may have worked out for best. According to the assessment of one of Dandy's successors at Hopkins, Dr. Donlin Long, "Had Dandy gone to Harvard, he would have undergone the traditional training program and followed the Cushing model. The losses to neurosurgery would have been great."[24] These words were written eighty-five years later.

Aside from the freedom for Dandy to develop professionally, the conflict with Cushing had no good results. Cushing was reluctant to accept the value of ventriculography, and those under his influence were reluctant as well. Neurosurgeons at the time were very polarized: either pro-Dandy or pro-Cushing, with the far greater number in the Cushing camp. Dandy, on his side, refused initially to join the Society of Neurological Surgeons, founded by Cushing, although he joined later.

In summary, Long concludes: "Cushing was the first neurosurgeon and established the field; Dandy was the first *modern* neurosurgeon, and his techniques are only now being supplanted through the use of magnification and technology."[25]

JOHN AND RACHEL DANDY IN ENGLAND AND IRELAND: **1911–1914**

While the conflict with Cushing was developing, John and Rachel were in England. The letters that went back and forth across the Atlantic provide insight to the extent to which all three were preoccupied with that conflict.

The trip (see Figure 2.18) was a voyage into their past. They visited family and friends in Barrow, Armagh, and Tarleton in England, and Bally Lane in Ireland. They attended church, went to meetings of the Socialist party, and visited with friends and family in Tarleton and Barrow in England,.

In November 1911, John wrote to Walter that "in the latter part of this week she [Rachel] is going to take and show me in Ireland those big hills she used to run down when a little girl. And the boys run [sic] after her. And she run away like she did from me on Bath Street [in Barrow]. She is feeling good and quite saucy and bossey. And looks fine in her new costumes."[26] A few days later, still in Ireland, he mentioned the schoolhouse "where the teacher could not teach her any more...Then we passed another school where she was whipped for talking (asking her brother for something to eat.)"[27]

John reveals himself as a very warm person, who responded to the Irish relatives. He was amused to note that Rachel's relatives thought he was very rich.

In their letters, both parents express their great love for their son and their pride in his accomplishments.

One letter comments on the sinking of the Titanic. Another event in the outside world was to influence them even more. Although they had entertained the idea of tak-

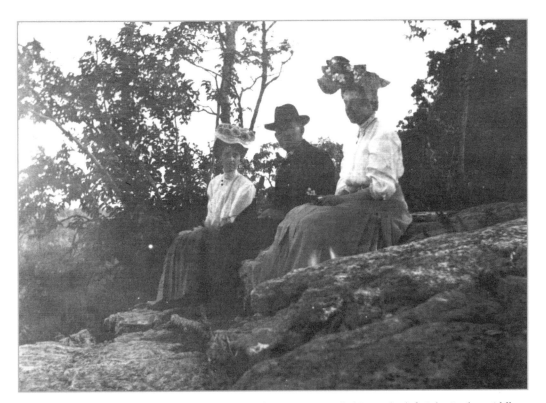

FIGURE 2.18 Rachel and John on an outing in the country. Rachel is on the left, John in the middle, and an unidentified friend on the right.

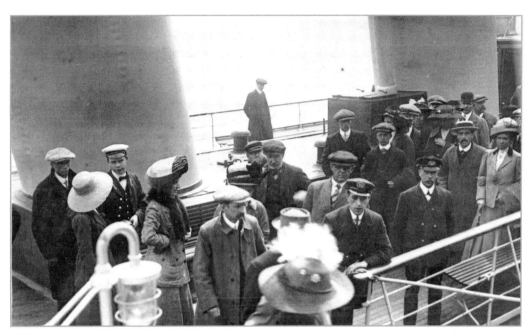

FIGURE 2.19   Rachel on the excursion boat to the Isle of Man, in the Irish Sea. She is on the left with the big hat, her hands on her hips, looking at John in the center of the picture dressed in a light colored suit and cap, July 13, 1912.

ing up residence in England, the prospect of war ended that. On August 16, 1914, Walter wrote his parents, "But another thing I want to know is whether you would object to me joining the Red Cross Corps for service in Europe. It will be a wonderful experience, a bully trip and will make $250 a month, see all Europe with all expenses paid and be entirely out of danger. Only Americans can serve, they are accepted by all combatants and they are out of line of danger entirely. I would get lots of war surgery to do, but the experience would be wonderful in every way. A number of men here are going at the first opportunity. I know you will think at first that it is war and will look at it like swimming but there isn't any more danger than there is with swimming. Everything is out of the way of the combatants. You can serve for 6 months or longer. Six months would be all I would want. It is the experience of a lifetime."[28]

For reasons that are lost to history, Walter did not join the Red Cross Corps. The letter, however, illustrates his lifelong attraction to adventure. Even as a young boy, Walter was not averse to risk–despite his mother's well-founded concern. The reference to swimming harkened back to boyhood days when he and his friends would hike some distance from Sedalia to swim in a local creek. There were other escapades to give his mother ample cause for concern as well. Memorable events included a near-miss of his head when his hunting rifle discharged while he was crawling under a fence, and plunging into the frigid waters of Fisher's lake near Sedalia while skating on thin ice. Walter's love of action and adventure continued throughout his life.

Once his parents had decided to return to Baltimore, Walter wrote them, "I have a beautiful house picked out for you and some furniture ready for you."[29] They returned to Baltimore in October of 1914. We assume that they took their son's advice to take the Pullman (first class) from New York and to buy a *New York Times* to read on the train.

JOHNS HOPKINS HOUSE STAFF VACATIONING ON THE EASTERN SHORE OF MARYLAND.

Figures 2.20–2.26 were taken at Clairborne, Maryland on the Eastern Shore of Chesapeake Bay.

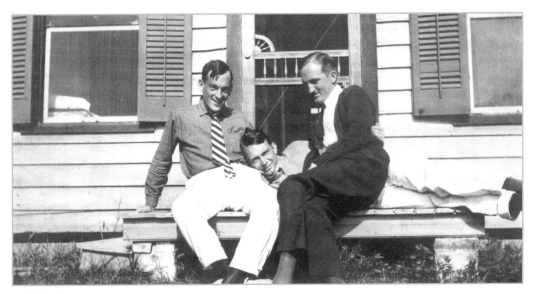

FIGURE 2.20   "Trying to be lazy" Dandy is in the middle.

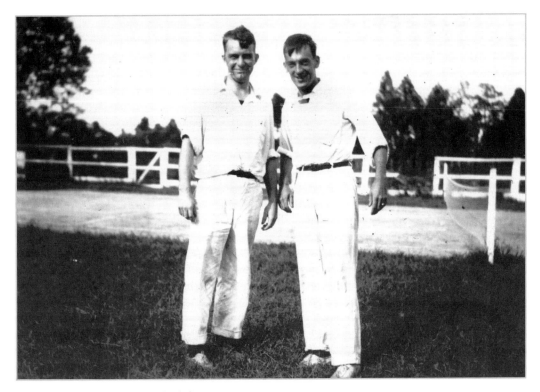

FIGURE 2.21   Dandy is on the left.

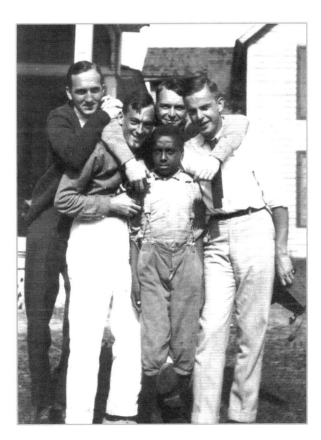

FIGURE 2.22   Dandy is in the center behind the child.

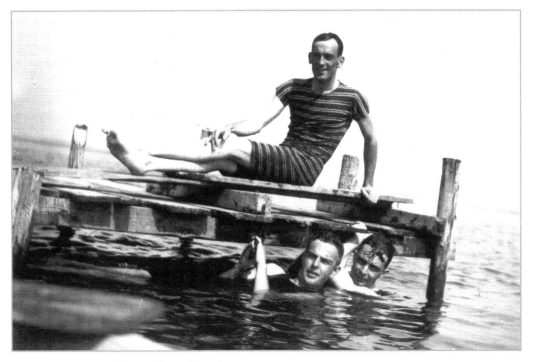

FIGURE 2.23   Dandy is on the right in the water.

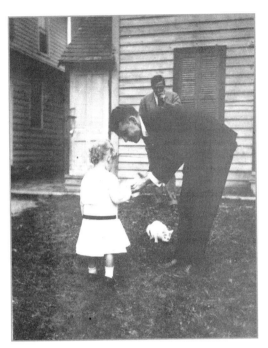

FIGURE 2.24 Dandy washing child's hands after he had touched a cat.

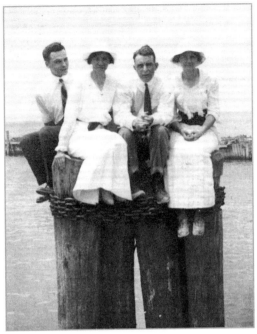

FIGURE 2.25 Dandy, second from the right, with friends.

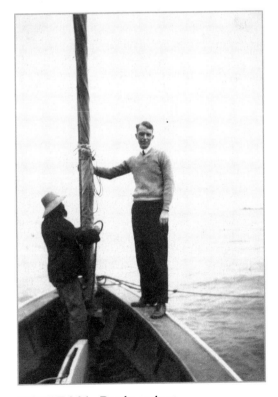

FIGURE 2.26 Dandy, on boat.

JEKYLL ISLAND: "DOCTORING IN PARADISE"[30]

One of the unexpected delights of this biography project was the view that has emerged of a vanished way of life. Nowhere is this more evident than in the scene of Jekyll Island,[31] a winter playground for the very rich off the coast of Georgia.

> "For 30 glorious winters starting just before World War I, a string of handpicked Hopkins physicians traveled south to tiny Jekyll Island off the coast of Georgia to tend to the ills and whims of 50 fabulously rich families. Jekyll . . . was the most elite, the most inaccessible private social club this country had ever known.[32]

Among the families who vacationed there were the Vanderbilts, Rockefellers, Morgans, Whitneys, and Astors. The wealthy families arrived by yacht and by train, usually in private railroad cars. While many members stayed in the club house (Figure 2.27), others built cottages for their family's winter visits. Less formal than the "cottages" at Newport where many of the families spent the summers, the houses were somewhat simpler, although one is reported to have had seventeen bathrooms!

Finding a physician for the club was not an easy matter, as the superintendent wrote in 1897. "One with a practice will not leave it, and one that is not good enough to get a practice in N.Y., we do not want here."[33] Several doctors from New York's Roosevelt Hospital, including Roy McClure, went to Jekyll. In 1912, when McClure went to Hopkins, Club officers wrote to William Halsted, Hopkins' Chief of Surgery, requesting that McClure be sent again, this time from Hopkins. Hopkins physicians became the "treaters of choice" for the wealthy club members and their guests.

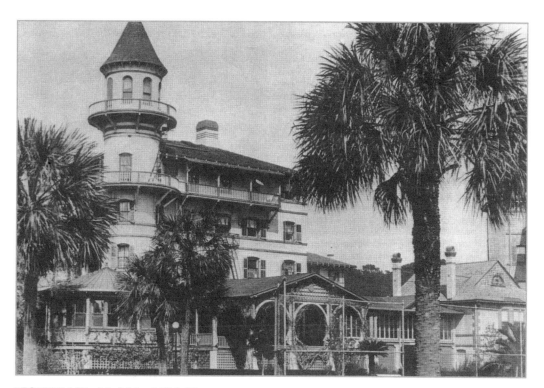

FIGURE 2.27   Jekyll Island Club House.

In 1915, after McClure left Hopkins, Halsted assigned his young resident Walter Dandy to serve at Jekyll for the winter seasons, often February through April. Dandy served for six successive seasons, and later described the "wonderful vacation Jekyll Island forces upon everyone who is fortunate enough to go there. I cannot tell you how much I have missed it and I am always trying to maneuver an opening so that I can again renew my old acquaintances and play around the wonderful golf course, swim and tennis."[34]

In January 1923, Dandy wrote to his parents about the winter at Jekyll (Figures 2.28 and 2.29), expressing his guarded enthusiasm for life among the wealthy. It is not hard to imagine what this young man, less than a decade away from his modest home in Sedalia, must have thought of the lifestyle at Jekyll. Resort life and that of his immigrant parents presented a great contrast. We detect a note of self-justification, if not apology, "I'm just beginning to appreciate fully the value of such a trip. A vacation like this means a great deal to a fellow who has been living in Hopkins Hospital for eighteen months. . . . The golf lessons are a daily exercise, although I've not yet gone around the course."[35] Despite his slow beginnings on the golf course, Dandy won a silver cup for golf. The cup graced the china closet in the dining room after his marriage.

Dandy's successor at Jekyll was his colleague and long-time friend, Warfield Firor, who served at Jekyll for 17 winters. Many of his patients "had fashionable doctors in New York who really didn't take care of them. They would send for me to come up to New York to advise them."[36] Many of the club members became patients at Hopkins and donated large amounts of money to the hospital.

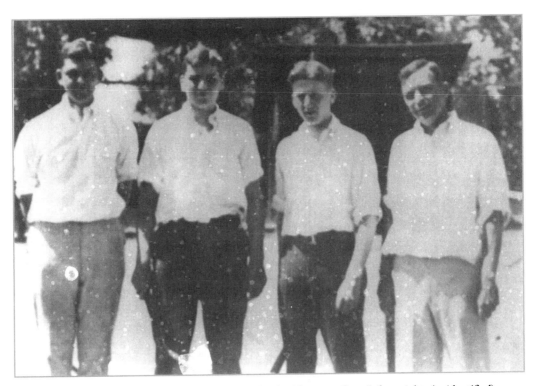

FIGURE 2.28   Dandy on tennis court at Jekyll Island with guests from left to right: (unidentified), Fuller Albright, John Joseph Albright, Jr., and Walter Dandy.

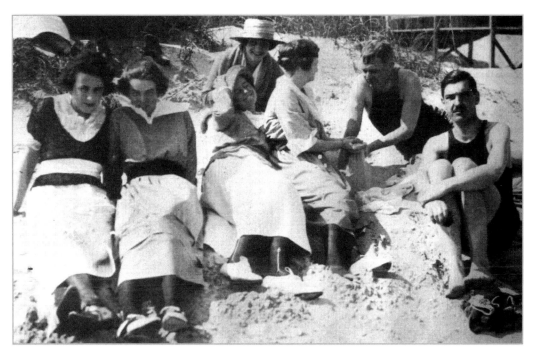

FIGURE 2.29   Dandy, second from the right, on the beach with the Roosevelts.

SUMMARY OF THE EARLY PROFESSIONAL YEARS: "DANDY WILL GO FAR"

At the end of this period, Dandy's course was set. He had graduated from college, completed medical school, and served as intern and resident under Dr. Halsted. His work on hydrocephalus and ventriculography was a major career development, for which he was recognized both in the United States and in Europe. In fact, he was nominated for a Nobel Prize for this work. Beginning in 1919, Dandy had offers from other medical institutions including Baylor and Vanderbilt. He decided to remain at Hopkins (Figure 2.30), and, in 1921, was appointed Associate Professor of Surgery in the medical school, and Assistant Visiting Surgeon at the hospital with a developing private practice.

In 1918, Halsted wrote to William Osler, then Regius Professor at Oxford:

> We miss him (Cushing) greatly although Dandy has developed remarkably. He gave by invitation a résumé of his work, experimental and clinical, on hydrocephalus at the semiannual meeting in Baltimore of the National Academy of Sciences. His contribution was quite unanimously pronounced the most important of the session. Dandy "will go far" as Welch says. I wonder if you have seen any of his papers. His pneumo-ventriculography has already proved of great value in the diagnosis and location of brain tumors as well as in the determination of the size and shape of the ventricular cavity. Dandy's father was until his recent retirement, a railroad engineer. Like most of the best products of Johns Hopkins Hospital, he comes from the west.[37]

Halsted died in 1922. Dandy had been very attentive to him when his health was failing, occasionally driving him around Baltimore.[38] After his death, Dandy wrote to Mrs. Halsted:

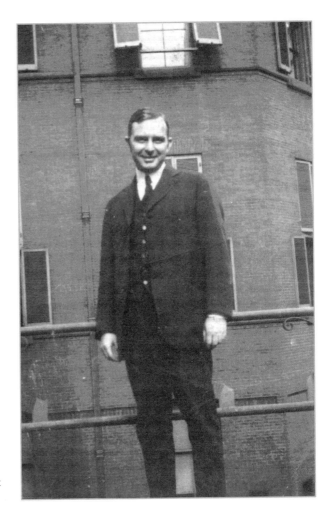

FIGURE 2.30 Dandy on the bridge at Hopkins about 1920.

> Dr. Halsted's loss is felt more keenly every day. I find myself constantly wishing to run up to his office to consult with him on new problems, a source from which I could always receive stimulation and at the same time modulation. His services can never die and to men who have worked with him, the stimulus will go on as long as they live.[39]

Also in 1922, Dr. J.M.T. Finney was appointed the new Chief of Surgery. Dr. Finney appointed Dandy's first full-time resident, Frederick Reichert, who became a lifelong friend.

The next year in Dandy's life was to be a very significant one.

Walter Dandy: Commentary on the Hopkins Years

By Donlin Long, M.D.

Walter Dandy was born in Sedalia, Missouri, the son of a recent immigrant railroad worker. Sedalia was then a major point on the MKT (Missouri, Kansas and Texas) railroad, affectionately known as the Katy. The elder Dandy was an engineer on that railroad; a well-paying job at the top of the blue collar chain. The Dandys were members of a radical left labor political group before they left England, and it can be assumed that the Dandy parents retained these political views in their new home.

Sedalia is about 40 miles from my home town of Jefferson City and about 70 miles from the home of the University of Missouri in Columbia where Dandy went to College. My first contact with Walter Dandy occurred in the gymnasium of the Smith-Cotton high school, the site of Walter Dandy's alma-mater. There, on the wall, was a black-and-white photograph of Dr. Dandy with the following inscription, "Walter Dandy, physician, said to have practiced in Baltimore."

Following high-school, Walter Dandy enrolled at the University of Missouri in Columbia. He was a good athlete, played center field on the Tiger baseball team and his behavior earned him the nickname "Roughneck." He entered the University of Missouri Medical School. My second encounter with Walter Dandy occurred on my first day of medical school in Jackson Hall. The professor of anatomy began our orientation by pointing his finger at me and loudly asking "Young man, do you know whose seat you're in?" Obviously I did not, but before I could respond, he proceeded to tell me and the class that I was sitting in the seat occupied by the great Walter Dandy, whose contributions he detailed for us as inspiration for our own careers. We were also shown the pathology drawings made by Dr. Dandy as a second year student as examples of what we should do in the same class. I later encountered the majority of the drawings in the collection at Johns Hopkins. Dr. Dandy was a remarkable medical artist and these drawings demonstrate that talent.

Walter Dandy completed his medical education at Johns Hopkins. At the University of Missouri, he had been a stellar student, excelling at every level. There is evidence from his letters to his parents that his first year at Johns Hopkins was not a particularly happy one. He had some scholastic problems while adjusting to the new environment and wrote to his parents about them. In answer, he received unfailing support which continually reinforced the idea that he was the best.

When Dandy arrived in Baltimore, Harvey Cushing's career in neurosurgery was blossoming. The Hunterian surgical research laboratory had opened a few years earlier with Cushing as its first director. His famous monograph on neurosurgery had been published in Keen's Practice of Surgery and his surgical practice was expanding. In those days, the Hunterian laboratory was managed by a Hunterian fellow. That fellow managed the laboratory, Cushing's research, and the surgical anatomy courses, as well as the animal hospital. Walter Dandy accepted this position in 1910. Thus, he became involved in Harvey Cushing's research. What began as a collaboration between a brilliant, young faculty member and surgical intern became one of the most famous confrontations in medical history. During his time at the Hunterian with Cushing, Walter Dandy studied the pituitary gland and its critical role in hormone production and imbalance. He also studied the pineal, and he developed the technique for experimental removal of both organs. He began a series of studies of spinal fluid production and experimental hydrocephalus, which would make him famous. It is interesting to note that Cushing and Weed wrote a series of collaborative papers on this work after Cushing left Johns Hopkins. Walter Dandy's name is absent from those publications and Dandy never included Cushing or Weed in his famous papers, either. Given the assignments at the time, it is impossible to believe that these had not begun as collaborative projects which the confrontation separated.

The origins of the famous Cushing—Dandy controversy will probably never be fully understood and the specifics are not known. However, the Dandy letters to his parents contain great insights into the origins of the quarrel. Dandy's letters consistently report to his parents that Dr. Cushing is rarely in the laboratory, that the ideas are mostly his (Walter Dandy's), and that the performance of the experiments is possible only because of his skills. He reports that Cushing drops into the laboratory to see

Continued

what he is doing. Cushing's major contribution is to opine that the experiment Dandy proposes is not technically feasible, and then Dandy triumphantly reports to his parrents that, a few weeks later, Cushing returns to see the finished experiment that Dandy has independently completed. We can presume that Harvey Cushing's view of the situation may have been very different. After all, he was a faculty member, director of the laboratory, and responsible for surgical research at Johns Hopkins, the fundraiser who made the Hunterian laboratory possible, and had been involved with the pituitary project before Walter Dandy assumed any role in the laboratory. thus, we have the controversy in progress with Dandy, a talented young intern who clearly believed that the Hunterian laboratory and its research are his, and an established faculty member who probably sees Dandy as only one of the progression of equally talented interns. but I believe the controversy is more subtle than this obvious, direct clash of realities. Cushing was a patrician from an eminent medical family, and Ivy League educated. Walter Dandy was from a blue collar, midwestern background with a base in radical, liberal, labor political thinking. both men recognized their own worth and a philosophical as well as practical confrontation seems to have been inevitable.

When Cushing accepted the newly created chair of surgery in Boston, it was assumed that Dandy would with him. The clash of personality, focused by Cushing's plan to take all the data from the Hunterian laboratory with him to Boston as his own property, led to the withdrawal of the offer to Dandy and left him without a position. Halsted was already gone for the summer and could not be contacted, so the director of the hospital took it upon himself to offer Dandy a non-paying research job with the virtual certainty that Halsted would provide a place for him in the surgical training program upon his return to Baltimore. Thus, Dandy began the superb research on the circulation of the spinal fluid and hydrocephalus, which many regard as the best surgical research ever done even today.

Dandy then did become a member of the surgical house staff. While a student and fellow, he had explained hydrocephalus and the circulation of the spinal fluid, topics which had frustrated the greatest pathologists and anatomists for hundreds of years. During his residency, he invented air encephalography. For the first time it was possible for the neurosurgeon to localize pathology before subjecting the patient to craniotomy. This great advance also led to the founding of the entire field of neuro-radiology. Some have described this as serendipitous. Dandy's writings at the time make it clear that he had a thorough philosophical conviction that imaging to localize pathology in the nervous system was required to advance the field.

Dandy completed surgical training in 1918. He joined the faculty as the only dedicated neurosurgeon and a member of the part-time faculty as Harvey Cushing had been.

The part time - full time system at Johns Hopkins requires some explanation. During Walter Dandy's time, most of the faculty were part-time. That is, they devoted their clinical practice to Johns Hopkins but remained in a private relationship with patients. Some received token payment from the institution, but most donated their time to teaching and research. Walter Dandy continued this tradition, and there was no full time (that is, full salary) neurosurgeon at Johns Hopkins until A. Earl Walker succeeded Dr. Dandy.

Very shortly after he became a faculty member, Dandy published a landmark paper in the *Journal of the American Medical Association* on the treatment of brain tumors.[1] In it, he championed surgery for cure and derided the Cushing concept of palliation on which Cushing had built his career. It was audacious to say the least. A young faculty member at Johns Hopkins was attacking the entire philosophy of the most powerful surgeon in America, perhaps in the world. Yet, time has proven Dandy right, and it is he who can claim to be the philosophical father of modern neurosurgery.

These philosophical concepts include accurate preoperative and intraoperative localization of pathology, and surgery for cure as fundamental precepts. With these ideas, Dandy was the first to carry out effective surgical treatment for arteriovenous malformations and aneurysms of the brain. He developed the foundation for our modern concept of skull base surgery. He described the special require

Continued

ments of surgery within the ventricles. He developed the entire concept of functional neurosurgery for the relief of symptoms, such as epilepsy and movement disorders. He expanded our understanding of spinal diseases and clearly established the neurosurgeon's role in treating non-tumorous conditions of the spine. Much of modern neurosurgery is based upon this practical and philosophical construct, rather than the much more limited, tumor-related practice of Harvey Cushing.

Despite these achievements, Dandy remained outside the mainstream of neurosurgery of the time. He was not much interested in the political or administrative aspects of medicine. He did not believe in training large numbers of neurosurgeons. He believed that neurosurgery was an independent specialty but should remain grounded in surgery. He delighted in agitating Harvey Cushing, and his letters to his parents have several pointed references to "sticking up to the old man." Yet, there was nothing vindictive or malicious in these criticisms. They were based in his firm conviction that his brand of neurosurgery was the way of future and time has proven him right.

There is another aspect of Walter Dandy that persists in neurosurgical practice today —his remarkable work ethic. When I arrived at to Johns Hopkins in 1973, the senior faculty still remembered the great Dr. Dandy. I was regaled with stories of his remarkable clinical acumen and his dazzling surgical technique. Dandy kept cursory records and none was available by 1973, but Frank Otenasek, who was Dandy's associate for a few years, told me that the 500 case per year volume that we could count in the Hopkins records wasn't nearly enough. He estimated Dr. Dandy's output at at least 750 operations per year or more.

Walter Dandy was a true genius of medicine. Finding the treasure trove of letters which he wrote and received will provide much for future historians who will analyze them and their importance in American medicine. They give great insight into the background, education, and personality of this remarkable man. Dandy's life has not received the literary attention that his accomplishments deserve. After all, he elucidated one of the great enigmas of medicine, hydrocephalus, through brilliantly conceived surgical research, and proved more than anyone else that the Halsted—Cushing concept of the clinician-scientist could be a reality. He developed our entire concept of imaging for anatomical localization of intracranial disease, and his observations led to birth of the field of neuroradiology and the development of the extremely detailed methods for the visualiztion of the brain and the spinal cord which we now have. He understood that palliation was not enough and pressed for surgical techniques that cure the patient. He expanded our field into vascular disease, functional neurosurgery, and the spine. He established the current scope of our specialty. Accurate localization and surgery for cure or permanent relief of symptoms are both fundamental to the modern philosophy of neurosurgery.

Everyone in neurosurgery knows Walter Dandy, but I believe the Dandy legacy in the field is less appreciated than it should be. Today we all follow Walter Dandy, not Harvey Cushing. This work may help restore Dandy to his rightful place in the pantheon of neurosurgical gods. The family vignettes, letters, and photographs help us understand the forces which formed this unusual man to whom we and our patients owe so much.

Commentary Endnotes

1. Dandy, W.E.: The treatment of brain tumors. *Journal of the American Medical Association*, 1921.
2. Long, D.M.: The founding philosophy of neurosurgery in philosophy of neurological surgery. In Awad, I.A.: *Neurosurgical Topics*. Park Ridge, Ill.: American Association of Neurological Surgery, 1995.
3. Long, D.M.: The Moseley Lecture: Harvey Cushing, Walter Dandy, and the Role of Johns Hopkins in the Philosophy of Neurosurgery. Delivered 12/13/01 New Haven, Connecticut.
   AU: please cite endnotes 2 and 3 in the commentary section

CHAPTER 3

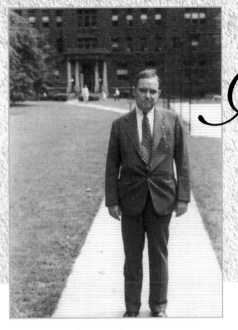

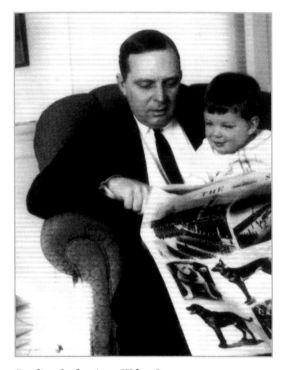

*M*arriage,
Family
and Career:
1923–1946

Dandy at Hopkins, 1936.

CHAPTER 3 OUTLINE

Reading the funnies to Walter Jr.

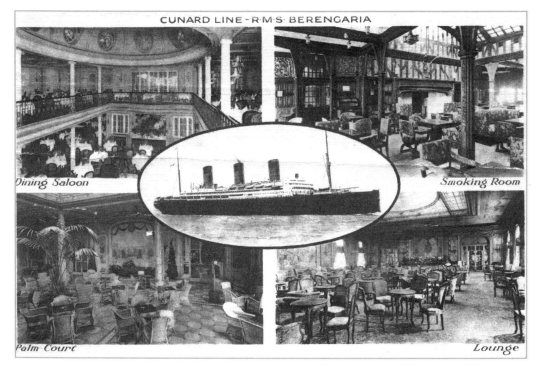

FIGURE 3.1   RMS Berengaria.

THE TRIP ABROAD

Walter Dandy made only one trip to Europe in his lifetime. He sailed from New York (Figures 3.1–3.3) in December 1923, with the intention of visiting European neurosurgeons and learning from them. Pediatrician Ned Park, a former Hopkins colleague, urged Dandy to go. Dandy secured a $10,000 education grant from the Rockefeller Foundation. His letters reveal his excitement in discovering what was to him, a new world of experiences in the "old world" of Europe, as he followed an itinerary of Paris, London, Paris, Amsterdam, Brussels, the Hague, Vienna, Munich, Berlin, Stockholm, Hamburg, Paris, Rome and Naples, Southern France, and London.

All but one of the surviving letters from this trip are to his parents in Baltimore. He also sent a letter and two postcards to Sadie Martin, a dietetic social worker at Hopkins, whom he had met in October, two months before sailing. He returned to Baltimore in April 1924.

In a postcard sent from the ship to Sadie, he writes:

> Ready to start. Such a wonderful boat! Looks impossible for any human means of forcing such a great thing ahead 3000 miles. Feel the thrill of a boy, but of course other emotions surge in too.[1]

The same excitement and enthusiasm pervades Dandy's letters to his parents. The following excerpts are from his letters to them and his letter to Sadie.

From Paris, the first stop, he writes:

> Here I am in this geese cackling place where I can't understand any more than Columbus understood from the Indians whom he discovered. The new year begins in Paris. It is a won-

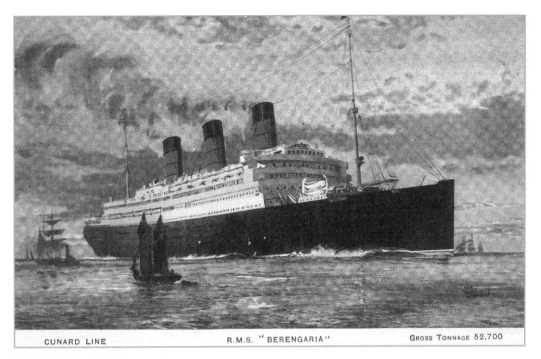

FIGURE 3.2   RMS Berengaria.

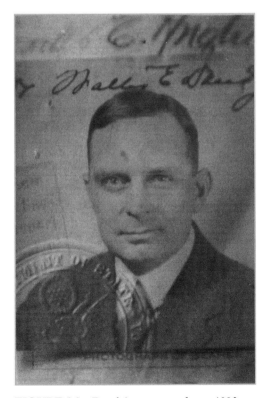

FIGURE 3.3   Dandy's passport photo, 1923.

derful city-as you of course know. Some of the most beautiful spots in the world are here. The Louvre is the finest art gallery in the world, includes all the finest paintings, etc., many of which were added by Napoleon. Napoleon's tomb is a very impressive thing. It is in the center of a great building. The sarcophagus is situated in a deep pit, mounted on a high pedestal. The Notre Dame Cathedral is the most wonderful building I have ever seen. It was 200 years in building, is entirely of stone, being built before the age of iron and steel. The great windows are said to be the finest. The great boulevards radiate out in all directions.

. . . a young French surgeon I met in Baltimore arranged to meet several doctors of the biggest reputations. They have been very good and eager to show me everything. The leading neurologist wants me to address the students in the University of Paris and they have asked me to operate. I have declined everything so far. Perhaps later I may on returning.

Every day brings new experiences and widens my horizon. Can't seem to learn any French but as there are so many English speaking people I get along satisfactorily. Haven't bothered about the loss of work as I expected I might.

From London:

What a beautiful contrast England is over France. Outside of Paris, France is a rather for-lorn looking place. The country from England's coast to London is so beautiful and well kept up, everything spic and span. It will be lovely in the spring. I shall hardly stay long in London and hardly do any sightseeing until spring when I return and when everything will be so much prettier.

Another doctor from Hopkins is going to Vienna with me and [will] stay as long as I do. I am not so sure how much work we are going to be able to get but we will see the world at any rate. So far I like America best.

I met a Baron and Baroness and they are surely nuts. No wonder Socialism grows in England. No human beings could be so inane. Let me know what you think of Miss Martin if she calls. I wrote her from Paris, thanking her for a little present (a book).

It is a fascinating city. I guess you have walked around everywhere. The first day I walked along the Thames to the Parliament building through Westminster Abbey, around Buckingham Palace into Piccadilly and down the mall into Trafalgar when it began to rain. Yesterday I tramped along the Bank of England, Cheapside, St. Paul's, Fleet Street, etc. . . . It's more fun wandering around at leisure here than anywhere I have been. Always some interesting historical old places come up when least expected.

I was much impressed with the English railways. They have doubtless improved a great deal since you were here. I, of course, have traveled 1st class. I could bet with a high degree of assurance what class you travel.

From Amsterdam:

Here I am in the most wonderful country in many ways that I have yet seen. It is such a beautiful thrifty country, irrigated through every few yards by ditches. The great windmills scattered everywhere and flapping their huge wings is a wonderful sight

Holland has been nice and clean and fairly cold just about freezing, but I have missed the good skating, which they usually have here most of the winter. This must be the place where the Dutch Cleanser got its name. You can't find dirt anywhere. It's a "spotless town" for sure. The buildings are all so beautiful, neat and tidy. The people dress so neatly and cleanly none of the slovenliness that I have seen in France, England and America. There seems no one very rich and very poor, but everyone in good circum-stances and well taken care of by their thrift. The people are all so open and friendly and kind. They go out of their way to help you for the love of doing it. They live sensibly. Not many motorcars. The cleanest little streetcars which move along at a snail pace, but you like it. Nearly everyone rides a bicycle. Holland is only about 25 miles radius from the center to the border and big thrifty cities are very close together. They have to speak German, English and French as well as their own Dutch because their neighbors are so close and they have to trade with them.

A month will have soon have passed. It won't be long 'til I'm back, but we won't "wish our lives away" will we? I wonder where I got that.

From Paris after his trip to The Hague:

The Hague with the famous Peace Palace is very beautiful and the city itself is very pretty. It is wealthier, but not quite so beautiful as Amsterdam, though both are so clean and beautiful.

I saw the most interesting work in Utrecht of anywhere. Professor Magussis is the principal light there and he was most thoroughly hospitable taking me to his home nearly every meal and spent his whole day doing nothing else than escorting me around and explaining in detail all that was going on. It was most interesting and will be useful. They were doing a lot of good work on the brain physiology in animals. There isn't much surgery of the brain there and I haven't been in the operating room yet. Perhaps on the return trip I will do more exploring of the surgical fields. Should have done so in England but the climate was so fierce, couldn't stand it.

From Vienna, after his thirty-six-hour trip from Paris on the Orient Express:

I am at the farthermost part of my journey. The Austrians are probably the best cooks in the world. The dinner on the diner was delicious. Much better than in France. . . . Shall meet Professor Eiselsberg one of the famous surgeons today

From Berlin, after Munich:

After three days in Munich I went to Zürich in Switzerland, again over mountains and across the very pretty Baden Lake for one hour. . . . Munich was very interesting both from a medical standpoint and from the view of the old city, where they make and drink so much beer. Have sauerkraut and wieners and pork and pig's feet and tripe-what a time Father would have floundering around in all of it. . . .

The best surgeon I have seen was in Munich and with it the finest experimental laboratory. -and not a full-time man, either. I have seen too much on my trip to ever think of full-time... It has been a very valuable experience, exactly opposite to what was expected. But I have to answer for myself and of course have no strings tied. I shall have to let the light shine slowly when I get back in order not to seem unappreciative. Have seen so much and learned so many new ideas that I shall have enough to do to keep me busy for a long time.

You will soon have the garden started. Don't work too hard in it! I hope you remain well.

From Berlin, he sent this letter to Sadie Martin:

At last, after traveling over most of Europe, your letter has just reached me. I had begun to think my friends had forgotten me. Wouldn't you have grand time in Europe? Paris, Vienna, London, Berlin. It would be a great inspiration to you. I know, to gaze on the wonderful displays in the windows during the day and such opera at night! And in Munich and Berlin, there is a great field for dietetic research on sauerkraut, pig's feet, pork and beer. Think what you could devise for your diabetic patients.

Such a wonderful place-Vienna-I could have stayed there 3 months instead of three weeks. They are such a cultured people. So kind and hospitable, you learn to love them more than any people you have ever met. The medical community and hospital far surpasses anything I have ever seen or imagined. And every night was the great opera (grand) with the world's finest orchestra. It was a difficult problem dodging entertainments by charming people to the even greater enjoyment of the opera. I could easily live without Paris or London, but not without Vienna. Berlin comes second: a greater busier city with great operas and art galleries and schools also. But there isn't quite the same feeling of an inbred culture, which [one] obtains in Vienna.

It has been a most agreeable surprise to find most Austrians and Germans without hatred. Among the official class of Germany, there is of course a latent hostility, mainly toward France, but principally to regain power. But the ordinary people are very different. They have suffered a great deal and are still, though less so. With wise leadership, they would be content to be at peace. But Europe is a great seething mass of politicians who use the people for cannonballs.

Today I visited the National Art Galleries-the finest collection of paintings-mostly German-many Rembrandts, too-I have seen far superior, I should say, to the great Louvre in Paris.

From Sweden:

We had a hard time getting here. We were 48 hours packed in the ice and couldn't budge until a warship broke the ice. Then we plowed through ice all the way to Sweden. The great Baltic Sea was frozen all the way across. It was a wonderful sight. I was the only one aboard who spoke English so I had to speak German. Sweden has mild temperatures compared to North Germany.

There is a good deal of snow here. I have just been out to watch them skiing. It is a wonderful and beautiful sport. A very vigorous climate makes a big strong nice people. Sweden is a lovely spot -much like England in the south: forests and mines in the north. There isn't much medical here, but it has been a wonderful trip. I enjoyed Berlin very much and liked the people except the ruling class.

From London:

Back in your old playground and I must say it looks better than any place I have seen. Surely it is the prettiest spot of all . . . I went on to Cardiff, Wales and, coming back, saw the first soil being turned over for gardens . . . Cardiff was on the sea and a little colder. It was beautiful country, all the way small farms and pretty hedges and trees. Everywhere it looked like a landscape artist had gotten there ahead and prepared everything in the most beautiful form.

From Paris:

There was a time when Paris seemed a long way from home. Now it seems quite near . . . Had a wonderful time in Rome and Naples, but I have had enough. The South of France is beautiful. It is still cool in Rome and in fact all Italy. The South of France alone is like spring, flowers out and gardens up.

Will you have some strawberries and onions for me when I get back? I am also hoping to be better received now than heretofore. Will you treat me better? I hope the car is all ready, too. I miss it very much. It will be good to be back again

Upon reflection of the trip, which came soon after World War I, Dandy concluded that American neurosurgical methods were, in general, more advanced than anything he had found in Europe. The friends he met there and the impact of European culture influenced the rest of his life.

His days as a bachelor would soon be over (Figure 3.4).

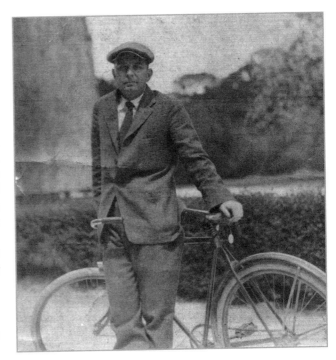

FIGURE 3.4 Dandy on a bicycle in the early '20s.

COURTSHIP AND MARRIAGE

Walter's courtship of Sadie had been interrupted by his trip to Europe. Sadie was an "old-fashioned girl" who wore her dark brown hair in a bun, not in a short bob like the flappers of the '20s (Figure 3.5). In later years, recalling the four-month separation, he would remind the children of that time by singing "My Bonnie Lies over the Ocean."

Because Dandy was considered a good "catch" by Hopkins employees, the courtship took place away from the hospital gossips. He courted Sadie in his prized car, a Wills Sainte Claire, taking her to football games in Annapolis and to dinner at their favorite Baltimore restaurant, Marconi's. At work, discretion

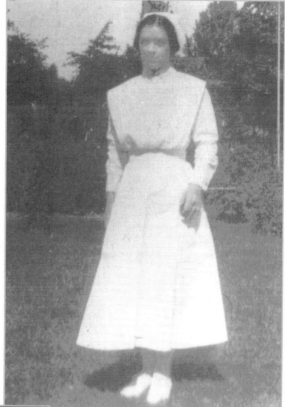

FIGURE 3.5   Sadie Martin, a dietician at Johns Hopkins.

was necessary. Sadie shared an office at the hospital with Emma Thomas, also a social worker. Emma later recalled hearing Walter's squeaky shoes as he approached their office, and a little behind-the-back wave he would give as he passed their open door.

On October 1, 1924, Walter Dandy and Sadie Martin were married at her family home on Sequoia Avenue in Baltimore (Figure 3.6). At the time of their marriage Walter was 38; Sadie was 23. They honeymooned for several weeks in the Adirondacks, canoeing and hiking (Figure 3.7). Even on his honeymoon, Dandy did not neglect his parents. He wrote: "The weather has been perfect, warm and clear. The coloring in the trees is gorgeous and to top it all, with the most wonderful little girl in the world . . ."[2]

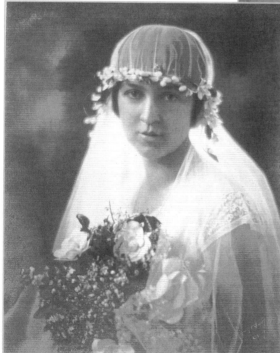

FIGURE 3.6   Sadie as bride, October 1924.

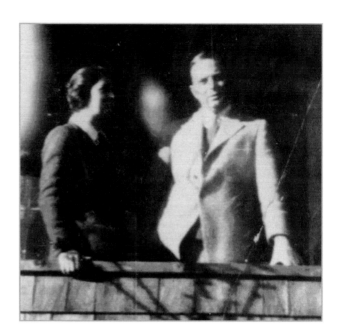

FIGURE 3. 7   The newlyweds in the Adirondacks.

STARTING A FAMILY: WALTER JR.

Upon their return to Baltimore, the newlyweds settled in the Temple Court apartments near Union Memorial Hospital. During their first year of marriage, they took a course in Art History at Sadie's alma mater, Goucher College, which they enjoyed. Dandy's enthusiasm for art had been discovered on his European tour and expressed in the letters to his parents. They also began planning their Georgian style house on Juniper Road in Guilford (Figure 3.8). The short fifteen-minute drive to the hospital was a major consideration in their choice of location.

In May 1925, Walter wrote his parents, "How fortunate I have also been in selecting my little girl. Few men have so much to be thankful for. She has been so sweet and unselfish and so eager to help. She seems so forgetful of herself. In many ways she makes me always reminiscent of my other little girl-who happens to be father's too."[3] He continued to call Sadie his "little girl" thoughout their marriage.

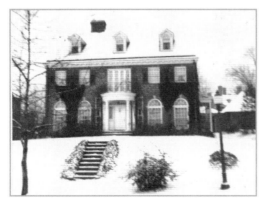

FIGURE 3.8   The Dandy house, 3904 Juniper Road.

On October 1, 1925, their first wedding anniversary, Walter Edward Dandy, Jr. was born at Johns Hopkins (Figures 3.10–3.14). When the new father first saw his baby, he burst into tears. He had seen so many ill or defective babies in his work that the sight of his own normal child was quite a relief.

Walter Jr. was described as "a handful," but his father would say, "Oh, he's just a boy."[4] When young Walter was eight months old, his father wrote, "How often I have seen the little rascal in my mind's eye and surveyed the beginning of intellect from the great mysterious void."[5] When little Walter was about two and a

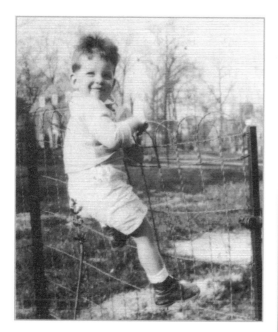

FIGURE 3.9   Walter Jr. on the fence at the new house, 1927. Walter's mother kept this photograph on her bureau.

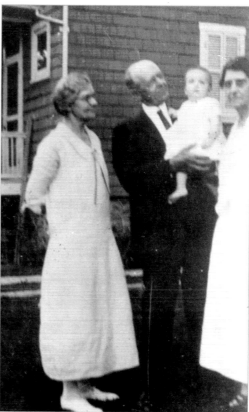

FIGURE 3.10   Walter Jr. with Grandmother Martin, Grandfather Dandy, and Grandmother Dandy, 1926.

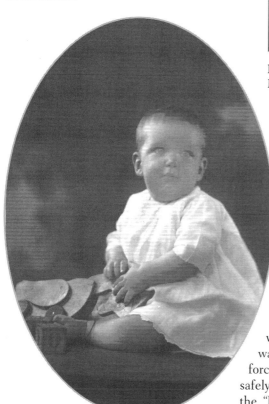

FIGURE 3.11   Walter Jr. in 1926.

half, his father wrote to his friend and former resident, Fred Reichert, that young Walter was "scampering all around the house and keeps his mother constantly on edge. He is just beginning to talk. It is a lot of fun watching his bright little mind develop."[6]

The three Dandys moved into their new home on Juniper Road in December 1926. It was designed for a family. The entry was a two-story hall with an encircling stairway. The banister on the stairway had been reinforced to allow future children to slide down safely. The backyard was completely fenced so that the "kiddies" could walk barefoot freely. The big open porch on the second floor was good for airing the little ones.

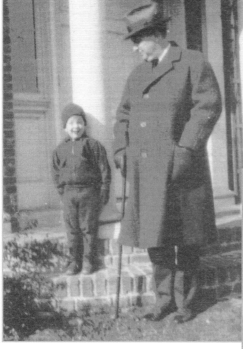

FIGURE 3.12   Walter Sr. off for a walk with Walter Jr. The cane had belonged to Dr. Halsted.

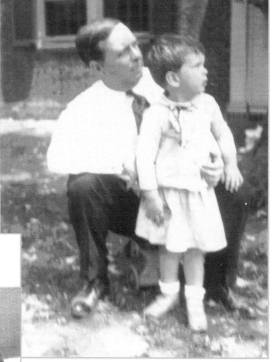

FIGURE 3.14   Walter Jr. in the dress his father had worn.

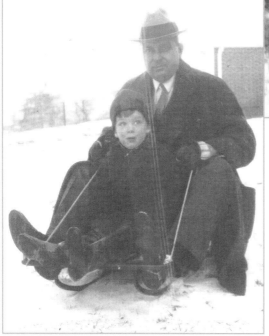

FIGURE 3.13   Sledding.

Mary Ellen

On July 22, 1927, the second child, Mary Ellen, was born (Figures 3.15–3.18). Like her brother, her hair at birth was red. Unlike her brother, whose hair turned brown, hers stayed red. Her father always said that if he had a beard, it would be red, but years later, when he caught the mumps from his youngest daughter, Margaret, the stubble that emerged was not red after all.

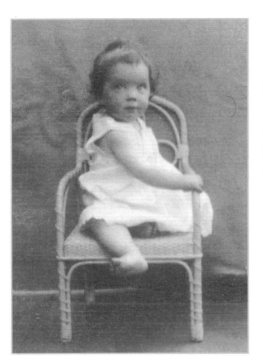

FIGURE 3.15   Mary Ellen, 1928.

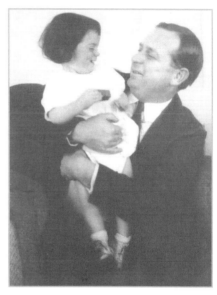

FIGURE 3.16   Mary Ellen and her father, 1929.

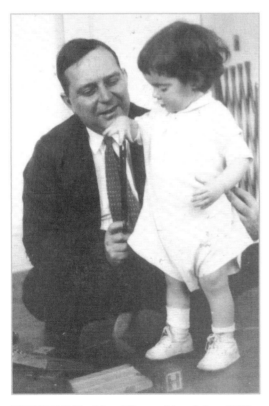

FIGURE 3.18   Mary Ellen and her father, 1929.

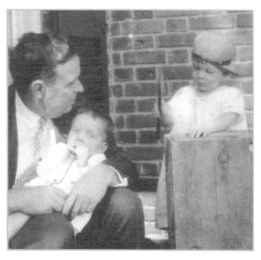

FIGURE 3.17   Walter Jr. with hammer, his father, and Mary Ellen, 1927.

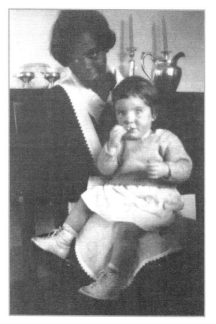

FIGURE 3.19   Aha holding Mary Ellen.

Shortly after Mary Ellen's birth, the Dandys hired a young woman, Helen Beatrice Davis, to do housework and child care. Helen came highly recommended by the mother of her "best beau," Weaver Dorsey, who had worked for the Martin family. The Dandy children called her Ha-Ha, which became Aha, a name that later even her friends used (Figure 3.19). Even after Aha and Weaver married in the mid '30s, Weaver was still called "Best Beau." The Dorseys had no children of their own, but Aha helped raise the Dandy children with the affectionate consistency she learned from her father, a Methodist minister. Weaver often took the Dandy children for rides in his grocery truck. He was a genial, fun-loving person, and both he and Aha were part of the family. Aha continued to work for "Miz Dandy" until the 1980s when they both entered retirement homes.

KITTY

On August 29, 1928, a third child arrived: Kathleen Louise, or Kitty Lou, as she was soon called (Figures 3.20–3.22). Kitty was an active, blond-haired baby who walked and talked very early and helped to turn the Dandy household into a very lively place. For the duration of one month-September-the three were only a year apart: Kitty was a newborn, Mary Ellen was one, and Walter, two. Their mother was probably exhausted.

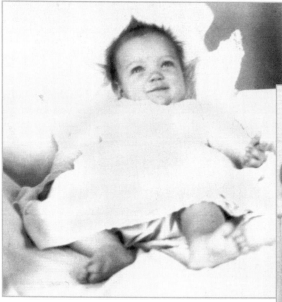

FIGURE 3.20   Kitty, 1928.

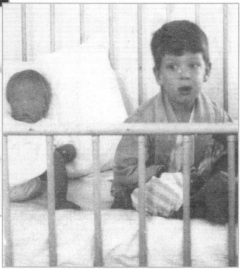

FIGURE 3.21   Kitty and Walter Jr., 1929.

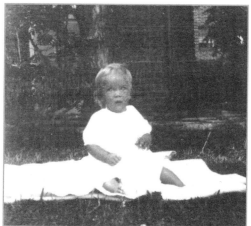

FIGURE 3.22 Kitty, 1929.

There was plenty of help. Assisting Aha in child care was a German governess, Hedel (Figure 3.23), and a succession of young black women. And there was a cook, Lily Gaines, a large black woman, who stayed many years with the family and provided them with food that was delicious, if unhealthy. (Traditional Southern cooking was high in fat, often bacon fat, and the vegetables were overcooked.) Sadie managed her "help" well, often encouraging them to continue with their education and helping the young ones with homework.

The Depression years had little effect on the family. Many years later, when Sadie was asked about the Depression, she could only remember that it prevented them from buying the property next door, out of fear that such a demonstration of prosperity might be resented by those less well off. The children did remember that when men came to the back door asking for handouts, they were given a sandwich, never money.

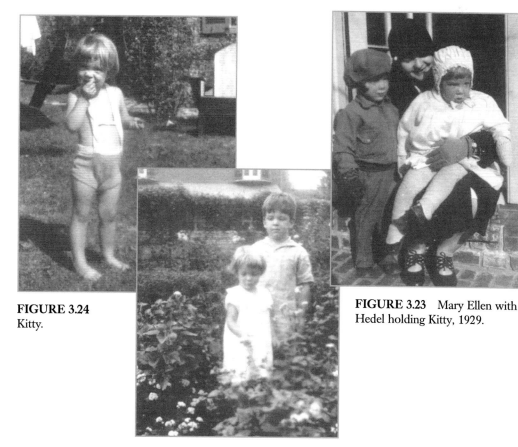

FIGURE 3.24
Kitty.

FIGURE 3.23 Mary Ellen with Hedel holding Kitty, 1929.

FIGURE 3.25 Walter Jr. and Kitty in the rose garden.

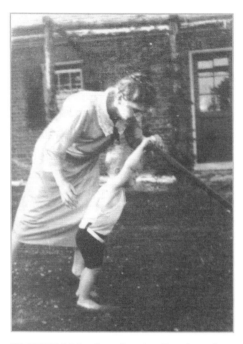

FIGURE 3.26   Grandmother Dandy and Walter Jr. mowing the grass.

LATE 'TWENTIES

Grandmother and Grandfather Dandy often came over to help the young family with carpentry and yard work (Figures 3.26 and 3.27). During the twenties and the ensuing Great Depression, Dr. Dandy continued his busy academic pace, writing thirty-four articles between 1923 and 1930. He also received an honorary degree (LLD) from the University of Missouri in 1928. Writing to Stratton Brooks, President of the University, to accept the honor, Dandy reaffirmed his ties to the institution: ". . . that the Honorary Degree of Doctor of Laws should first come from my Alma Mater will always be a source of even greater pride and satisfaction."[7] (Figure 3.28) He served on the board of trustees of the Missouri Medical School foundation, and for two years on an advisory council of the Board of Trustees of the University. He supported students of his former professor, W. C. Curtis, sending checks to some of the students Curtis took with him for summers at the Marine Biological Laboratory at Woods Hole, Mass.[8] Curtis and his

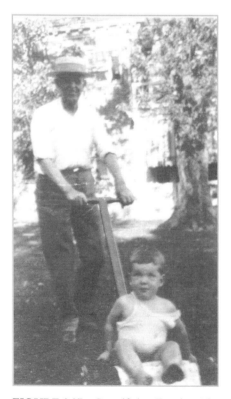

FIGURE 3.27   Grandfather Dandy with Walter on the lawn mower.

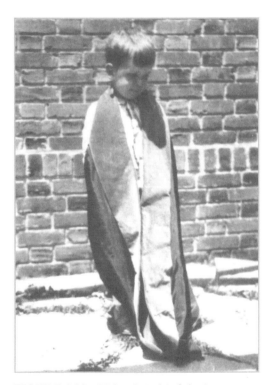

FIGURE 3.28   Walter Jr. in his father's academic hood.

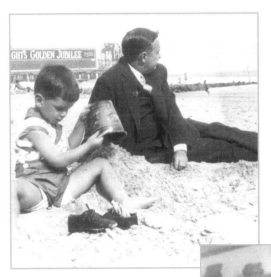

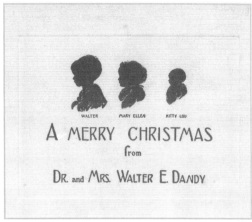

FIGURE 3.29   Dandy and his son at the beach.

FIGURE 3.30
The Dandy family
Christmas card,
1928.

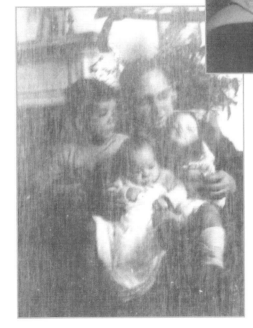

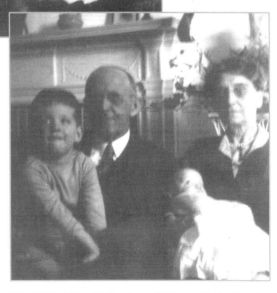

FIGURE 3.31
Dandy with Walter
Jr., and Kitty,
Christmas 1928.

FIGURE 3.32   Dandy and his three children, 1928.

FIGURE 3.33   Walter Jr. and Kitty with the Dandy grandparents.

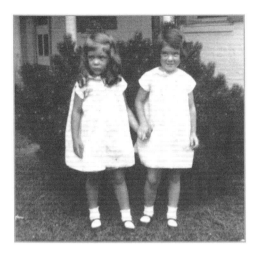

FIGURE 3.34   Mary Ellen and Kitty, 1933.

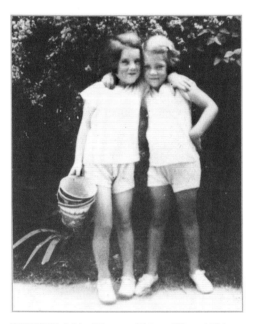

FIGURE 3.36   Kitty and Mary Ellen, 1934.

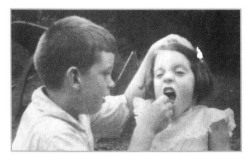

FIGURE 3.38   Walter Jr. pulling Mary Ellen's tooth.

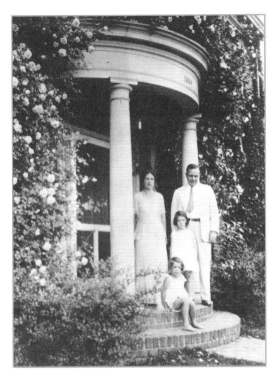

FIGURE 3.35   Sadie and Walter Dandy with Mary Ellen (standing) and Kitty (sitting) in front of the Juniper Road house.

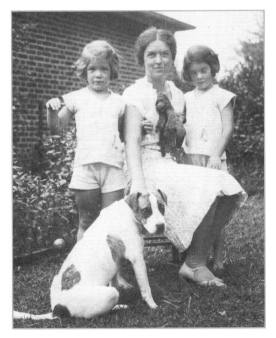

FIGURE 3.37   Kitty and Mary Ellen with their mother and their dog, Fagin, who was a gift from the Woodhalls.

colleague Lefevre, were important in Dandy's decision to go to medical school at Hopkins.

During visits to Columbia, Dandy often stayed with his old Sedalia friend, Stanley Battersby, now a Professor of Pediatrics at the University of Missouri. He was able to renew his acquaintance with some of his former professors, especially Winterton Curtis, but Professor Lefevre was no longer living.

THE DANDY HOME ON JUNIPER ROAD

Margaret

A new baby! Margaret Martin Dandy arrived on January 21, 1935 (Figures 3.39–3.44). The three young Dandys were completely surprised by Margaret's arrival. No one had told them anything about a baby! In those days, parents did not discuss such topics as pregnancy with children. ("None of the children ever asked" was the explanation.) Margaret was a plump, lovable baby. In the picture below, taken in the parents' bedroom, Dandy admires his newest child.

This bedroom held many memories for the Dandy children. On Sunday evenings, they would often climb onto the bed with their father to listen to radio comedians Jack Benny and Edgar Bergen with Charlie McCarthy. On warm summer evenings, they would hear the sounds of Orioles broadcasts from the radio. On other occasions, when he thought a head rub would relax him, their father lured them by promising money: 10 cents an hour for the head rub, and 25 cents if he fell asleep and stayed asleep while they slid off the bed. (These were Depression wages!) Another event that took place in the bedroom was the "trouser ceremony" [continue]

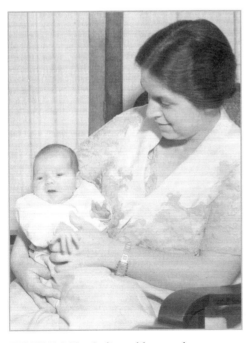

FIGURE 3.39 Sadie and her newborn daughter, Margaret Martin Dandy, 1935.

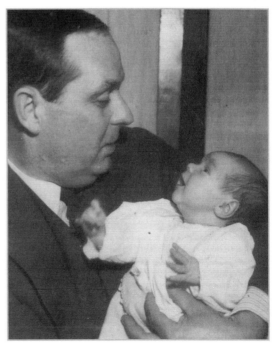

FIGURE 3.40 Margaret at 10 days old with her father.

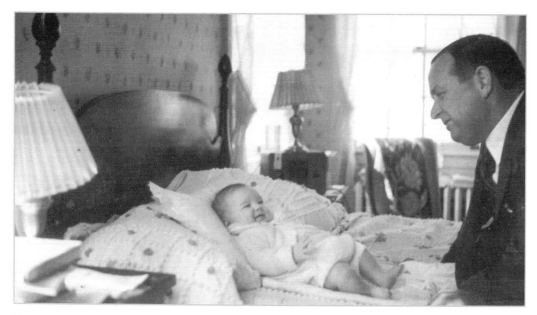

FIGURE 3.41   Dandy with his daughter Margaret, 1935.

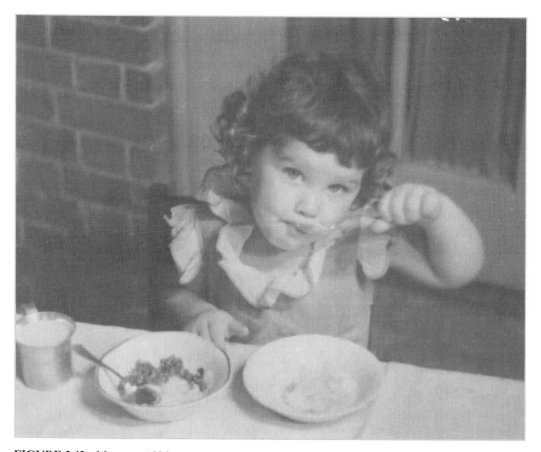

FIGURE 3.42   Margaret, 1936.

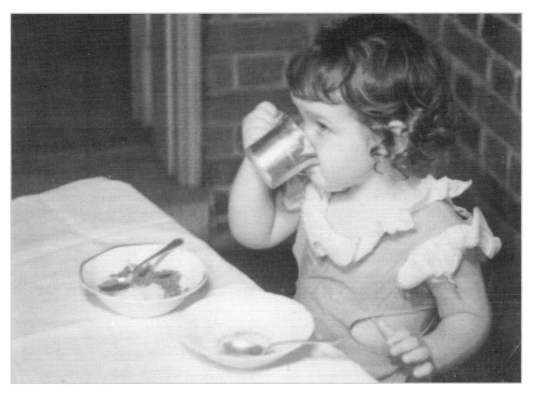

FIGURE 3.43   Margaret, 1936.

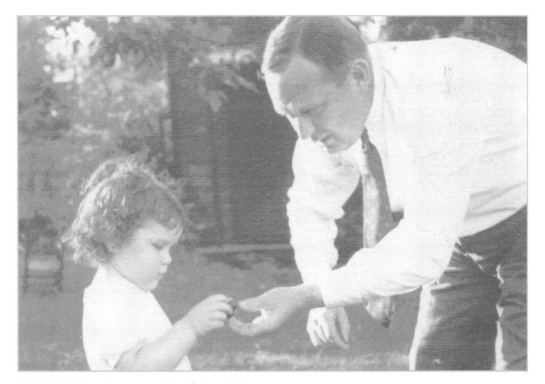

FIGURE 3.44   Margaret and her father, 1936.

at the end of the day. When Dandy turned his trousers upside down before hanging them in the closet, coins tumbled out. The children scrambled for the loose change, chanting "Finders keepers, losers weepers."

Another part of the bedroom that fascinated the children was their mother's closet. They loved to go into the closet and whistle down the tube to the pantry, where Aha would answer the call-1930s high tech!

When "Gangbusters" came on the radio and the "Ten Most Wanted Criminals" were read out, the older children huddled together on the big bed, fearful that one of the ten would be nearby. These were frightening times with criminal gangs. In 1932, when the Lindbergh baby was kidnapped, new locks were installed on the windows of the house. And then there was the gypsy queen who came to Hopkins for brain surgery with her entourage. At the time of the surgery, the gypsies pulled their mattresses from their big black cars, camped out, ordered food in local restaurants and left without paying, and were generally disruptive in the Hopkins area. When the gypsy queen died, the Dandys' fears increased. Like the imaginary kidnappers, the gypsies might be lurking nearby. Fortunately, the Dandy family was not bothered by the grieving gypsies, nor by the feared criminal gangs.

Summers in the '30s: Indian Landing

Baltimore summers are not always pleasant, although Walter Dandy never seemed to mind them. Sadie, who hated the heat and humidity, marveled that he could stand through four-hour operations with only fans to cool him, or play eighteen holes of golf and enjoy it! For the rest of the family, there were various escapes, near and far (Figures 3.45–3.52).

During the '30s, their mother drove the children through downtown Baltimore, past the ferry docks and the wonderful smells of the McCormick Spice Company (located near the present day Inner Harbor), and on to Indian Landing on the Severn River. Aha

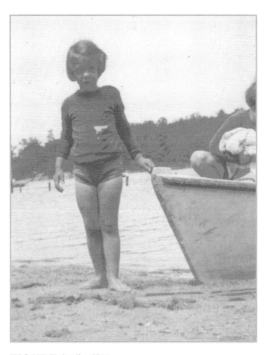

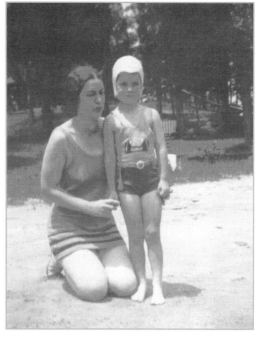

FIGURE 3.45   Kitty.

FIGURE 3.46   Mary Ellen and her mother.

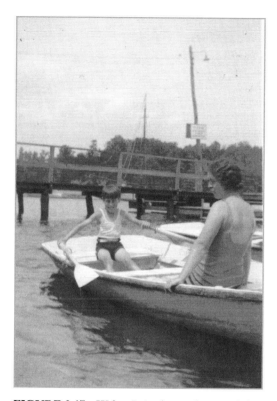

FIGURE 3.47   Walter Jr. in the rowboat with his mother.

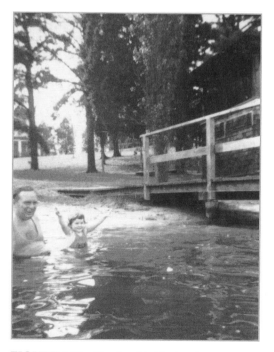

FIGURE 3.50   Dandy with his daughter, Margaret.

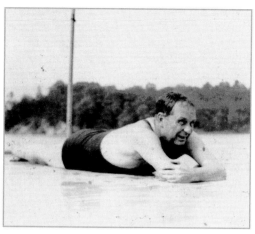

FIGURE 3.48   Dandy sunning himself on the raft.

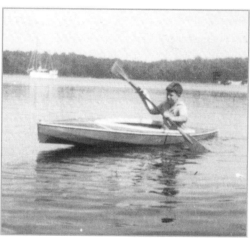

FIGURE 3.49   Walter Jr. paddling the kayak he built himself.

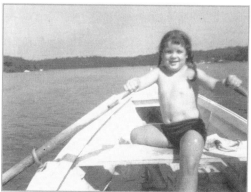

FIGURE 3.51   Margaret learning to row.

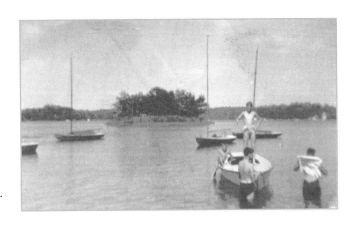

FIGURE 3.52 Walter Jr. and the sixteen-foot Comet sailboat he built.

packed a picnic basket that always included deviled eggs-each half wrapped carefully in waxed paper. She also sent along a big Thermos jug of lemonade. At Indian Landing, the children rowed boats and learned to swim. As they became stronger swimmers, they would swim to the "Little Island" where their mother's friend Emma Thomas often stayed in a small stone house. In August, the stinging sea nettles moved into the waters and swimming was less pleasant.

These trips to Indian Landing were enriched by the boats young Walter built: first a kayak, and then a sixteen-foot Comet sailboat. Both were built in the sunporch of the Juniper Road house, with encouragement from his parents.

SUMMERS IN THE '30s (VACATIONS AWAY)

Beginning in 1933, Walter Jr. went to Camp Gunston, on the Eastern Shore. His father kept up his habit of frequent letter writing. On July 22, 1933,[9] he wrote:

My Dear Boy:

Mother and I will probably be down to see you next Saturday. Do you want to stay another month or come home now. Let us know. We all want you with us but if you are happier at camp we can wait another month.

Mary Ellen had her birthday party yesterday at Indian Landing. She went in up to her neck. Kitty Lou turned a sommersault in the water. They have rubber wings! We heard that you are a very good swimmer now that you actually swam the river. That was difficult for us to believe. Also glad you had passed the canoe test and could dive. Fagin [family's English bull terrier] is getting so smart. He doesn't eat the newspaper. He plays with the little girls but I don't think he gets so much kick out of them for they don't quite know how to handle him like his boy friend. I am sure he will feel happier when you return. He has a little friend across the street. Every afternoon they meet on the lot and play.

Please write Grandmother and Grandfather Dandy a card-they are at 3021 ARUNAH AVE. It will make them very happy for they are always thinking about you. Tell them what you are doing and ask them to come to see you. Trusting you are having a continuous good time is my wish for you.

Daddy

Mary Ellen wants you to come home-also Kitty Lou.

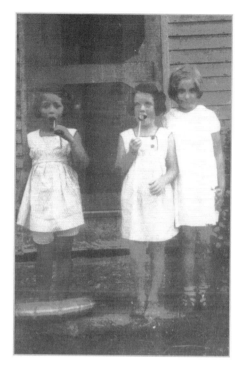

FIGURE 3.53 Kitty, Mary Ellen, and Connie Conradi at the farmhouse in Center Conway, New Hampshire, 1936.

With so much help at home, it was possible to leave Margaret behind for family vacations, because she was considered too young to participate in the activities. Pine Grove Farm in Raymond, Maine was one destination. The children remember their father sitting by the barn for what seemed like an hour watching a spider weave its web. He was actively observing, not daydreaming. The natural world fascinated him and he was a skilled observer. He owned the entire collection of Fabre's *Life of Insects*.

Walter Jr. continued at Camp Gunston until 1938, when he switched to Hyde Bay Camp in Cooperstown, New York with some of his school friends from Gilman School. Mary Ellen and Kitty went to Camp Marlyn in Andover, New Hampshire in 1939, then to Cloudmarch Camp in Damarascotta Mills, Maine in 1940. In 1941, Mary Ellen went back to Camp Marlyn and Kitty went to Pathfinder Camp, Hyde Bay's sister camp in Cooperstown, New York, in 1941.

In 1939, before the older girls went to summer camp, they went with their mother and father on a western trip: on the *Denver Zephyr* streamliner (train) to Denver, then on to Estes Park, and Yellowstone Park. Their father revisited some of the places he had seen in his trip after college.

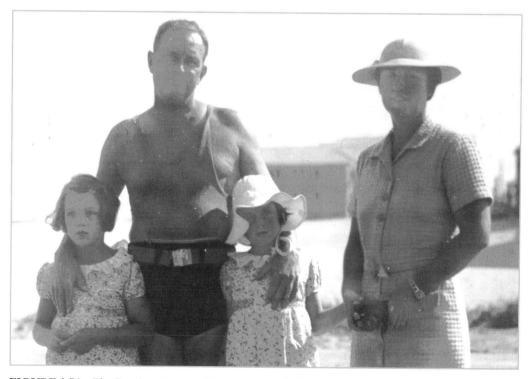

FIGURE 3.54 The Dandys at Ocean City, Maryland, 1935.

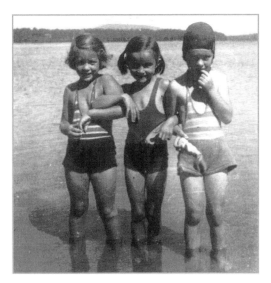

FIGURE 3.55   Kitty, Mary Ellen, and a friend at Pine Grove Farm in Maine, 1934.

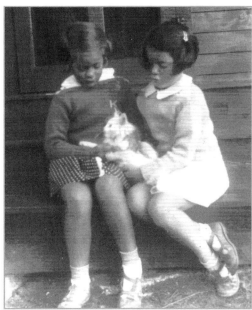

FIGURE 3.56   Kitty and Mary Ellen with a kitten in New Hampshire, 1936.

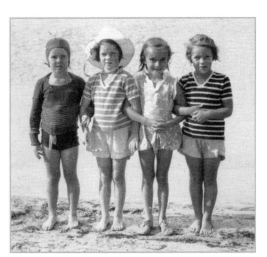

FIGURE 3.57   Mary Ellen and Kitty with friends at Pine Grove Farm, 1937.

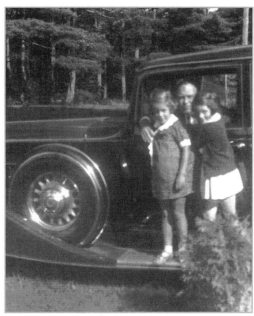

FIGURE 3.58   Kitty and Mary Ellen on the running board of their father's car at Pine Grove Farm.

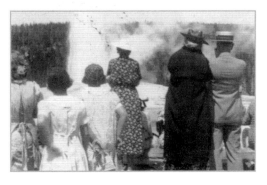

FIGURE 3.59   Kitty and Mary Ellen watching Old Faithful, 1939.

Summers in the '30s: Juniper Road and Nearby (Figures 3.60–3.65)

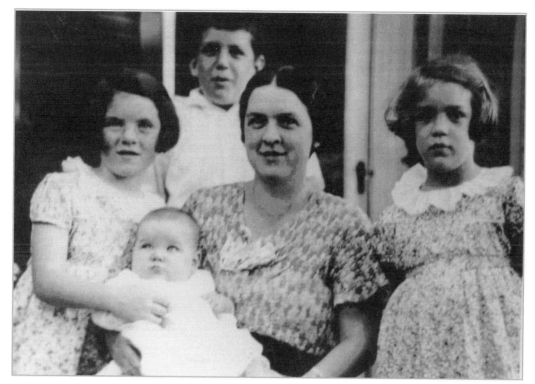

FIGURE 3.60 The Dandy children and their mother, 1935.

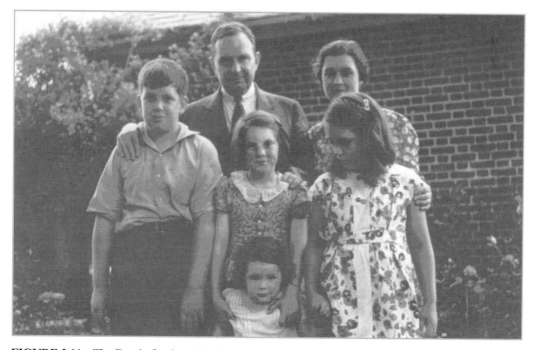

FIGURE 3.61 The Dandy family, 1936. This is the only existing photograph of the entire Dandy family.

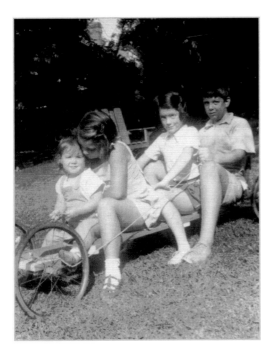

FIGURE 3.62   Margaret, Kitty, Mary Ellen and Walter Jr., on the cart that he built, 1937.

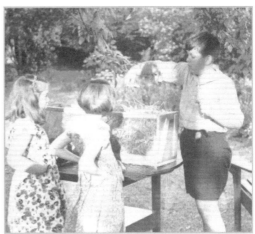

FIGURE 3.63   Walter Jr. showing his sisters his snake, 1936.

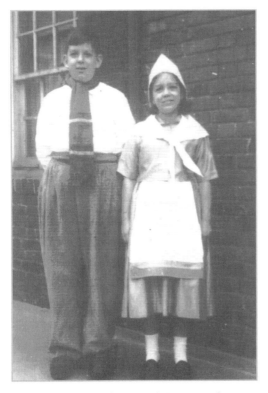

FIGURE 3.64   Walter Jr. and Kitty in a play at Calvert School.

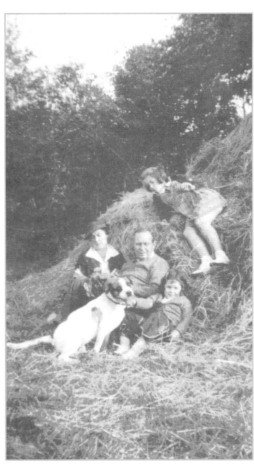

FIGURE 3.65   The Dandy family on a Sunday outing in the country.

Visiting the Grandparents

A Sunday ritual developed. Although Dandy seldom attended church, the rest of the family walked to the nearby Second Presbyterian Sunday School. On Sunday afternoons the whole family visited the grandparents (Figures 3.66–3.68). Stopping at the Martin house on Sequoia Avenue first, the children played the Victrola and helped Granddaddy Martin count the collection money from that morning's church service. From there the family went to the Arunah Avenue row house, home of Granddaddy and Grandmother Dandy. Granddaddy Dandy was often sitting by the window reading the Bible, and Grandmother Dandy was preparing the Sunday dinner-fried chicken, German-style potato salad, and fresh vegetables from John's garden. The small backyard was completely filled with his carefully tended vegetable garden, including grapes for wine. There were even chickens. Figure 3.68 shows young Margaret with some beets she had picked from the garden.

John and Rachel Dandy had lived in the house since their return from Europe in 1914. Rachel died in July 1936, at the age of seventy-five, of pneumonia. The news reached the family in New Hampshire when their father called from Johns Hopkins saying that his mother had just died. Mary Ellen remembers coming up the driveway and seeing her father cry when he met the family. It was the only time she ever saw him cry.

John Dandy lived on in the house and died in the Spring of 1940, shortly before his eighty-fourth birthday.

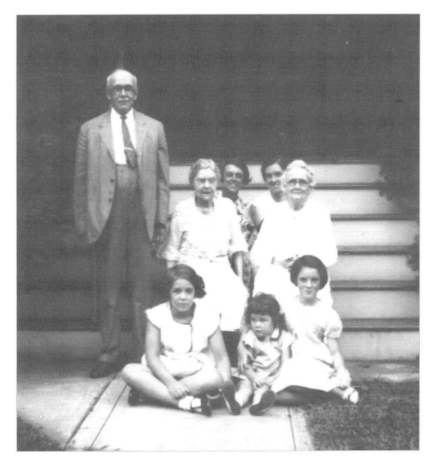

FIGURE 3.66
Visiting the Martin grandparents, 1936.

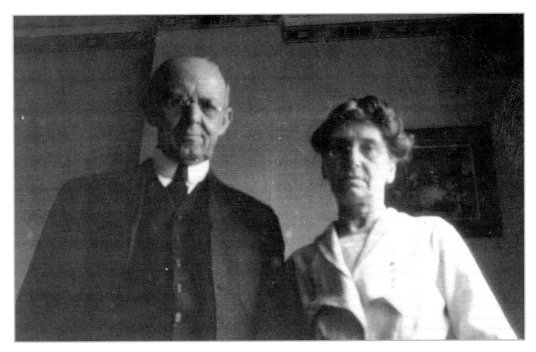

FIGURE 3.67   John and Rachel Dandy in their home in the 1930s.

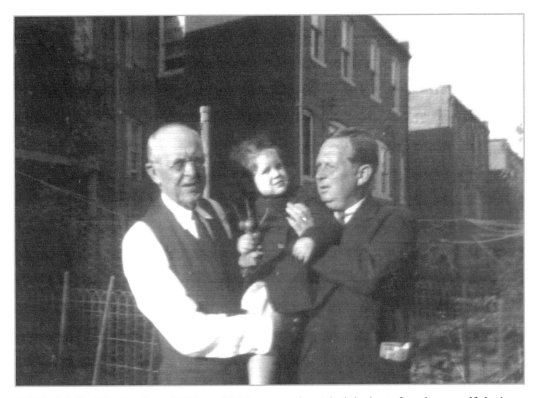

FIGURE 3.68   John Dandy and Walter with Margaret, who picked the beets from her grandfather's garden.

Brain Team

The practice of medicine during the '20s and '30s was quite different from today. Barnes Woodhall, M. D., a member of the Brain Team (Figures 3.69–3.71) from 1926–1937 describes the situation:

> Life expectancy for the male was 57.27 years, for the female 60.67. . . . Medicine was not an attractive career. Infection was everywhere and research was of feeble stature. . . . We lived with diphtheria, scarlet fever, meningitis, septicemia, typhoid fever, malaria, tuberculosis, gonorrhea, syphilis and post operative infection almost as bedfellows. Hospital mortality for even moderately severe infections was approximately 75%.[10]

Pressure in surgery was intense; tempers flared. Dandy was known for his temper in the operating room. There was no room for error. Woodhall recalls: "I was fired outright once and that held for only six hours."[11]

Brain surgery for Dandy was consuming, but it was also a team effort. He operated all day Tuesday, Wednesday, Friday, and Saturday morning, and he played golf on Thursday and Saturday afternoon. Dandy's faithful secretary, Bertha Schauck, scheduled all patients to be seen at noon in his office in the hospital. Members of the Brain Team included the chief resident, one or two assistant residents, an intern, and assorted nurses. The regulars on the team were Dandy's anesthetist, Grace Smith, his orderly, Lawrence, and his secretary, Mrs. Schauck.

For this highly productive surgeon, days were scheduled tightly to maximize the availability of the operating room. A typical day in the operating room is described in Appendix III: Walter Dandy – Super-Surgeon, by J. DeWitt Fox, M.D.

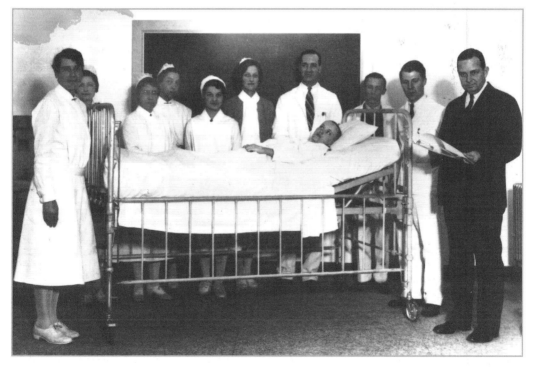

FIGURE 3.69 Dandy (at right) with members of the Brain Team in the 1930s. Barnes Woodhall is third from the right.

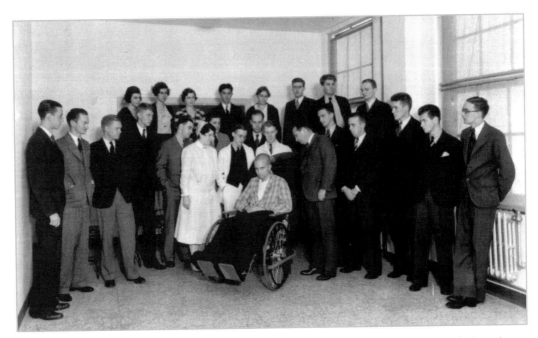

FIGURE 3.70 Neurosurgery rounds with the Medical School Class of 1933. Walter Dandy is to the right of the wheelchair, Barnes Woodhall is to the right of the nurse.

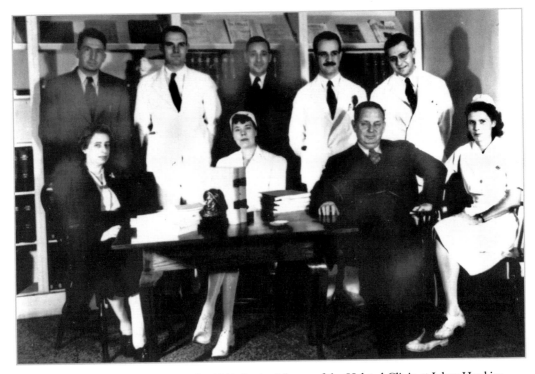

FIGURE 3.71 The Brain Team in the 1940s in the Library of the Halsted Clinic at Johns Hopkins. Back row, left to right: John Chambers, Charles Burkland, Frank J. Otenasek, Fermin Barcala, and Hugo Rizzoli. Front row, left to right: Mrs. Bertha Shauck, Dandy's secretary; Grace Smith, nurse anesthetist; Walter Dandy; and Miss Sarah (Susie) Lambert, scrub nurse.

Family Life Accommodates a Surgeon

At 7 p.m. every night, Dandy's chief resident would call him at home to report on the patients. (Sunday nights were the exception, because the family listened to Jack Benny on the radio.) The Dandy children often dialed the number "Wolfe five, five hundred." When the Hopkins operator answered, they were taught to ask "Would you have Dr. (the resident) call Dr. Dandy, please?" At other times, the children were cautioned against personal calls in case someone was trying to reach their father. Someone had to always be at home to answer the phone. When he took the children to the movies, their mother stayed home to answer the phone. These were the days before answering machines, voice mail, or answering services.

Dandy often discussed his surgeries at the dinner table, with vivid descriptions of the "beautiful" brain tumor he had removed that day. From the late '30s on, the older children occasionally visited the operating room to watch their father in action. From the gallery they could see him, brace and bit in hand, drill four holes in the patient's skull, use a flexible saw to cut between the holes, and remove the portion of skull to reveal the brain underneath. At times, their father would ask Lawrence, the orderly, to escort the visiting child to the floor of the operating room to a position behind him, where the child could get a better view and hear their father's narration of what was happening in the surgery.

The family participated in various ways at the hospital. In the late '30s, Sadie noted that the patients sat on stiff wooden benches as they waited for their appointments. She furnished a nearby spare room with comfortable furniture and a rocking chair for moth-

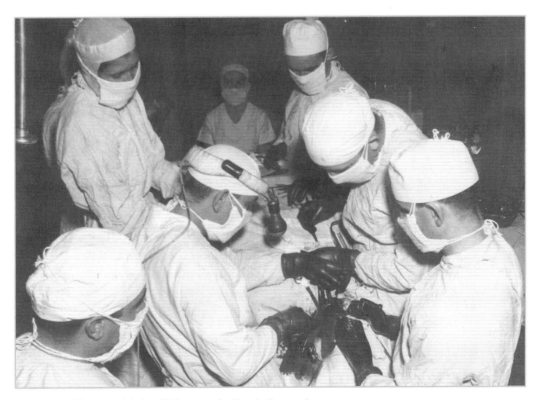

FIGURE 3.72   Dandy's headlight worn by Frank Otenasek.

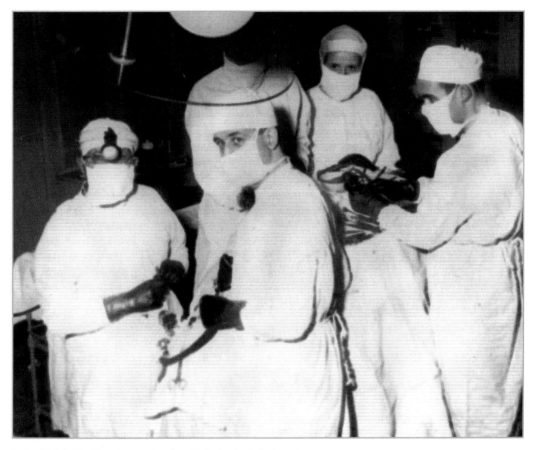

FIGURE 3.73   Dandy wearing headlight he had designed.

ers to rock their sick babies. The two older girls broadened their experience by working in the hospital during the summers. Beginning in 1943, Mary Ellen assisted Mrs. Schauck in her office and acted as a "receptionist" with the patients. The images of mothers carrying their hydrocephalic babies in their arms were never forgotten. Kitty helped in a clinic that served pregnant women and young girls. Most were poor; many were unwed. Kitty also remembers a young German prisoner of war scrubbing the hospital floors. Through his teenage years, young Walter often watched his father operate on Saturdays and learned how to develop film while working with Mr. Mann, the hospital photographer. When he began Medical School at Hopkins in 1944, he rode with his father to school every day, until his father's death in April of 1946.

When the children observed in the operating room, the atmosphere wasn't always serious. More than once their father would call out "Lawrence!" in a particular tone of voice. Lawrence knew the tone; it meant that it was time to hike up Dandy's trousers to a more secure position around his waist.

In the '40s, Walter Jr., a student at Hopkins Medical School, attended Harvard Medical School for a term. When he was observing in the gallery of the surgery operating room, Walter was introduced to the man standing next to him as Walter Dandy. With a twinkle, the man replied: "Yes, and my name is Cushing." (Cushing had died several years before this event.)

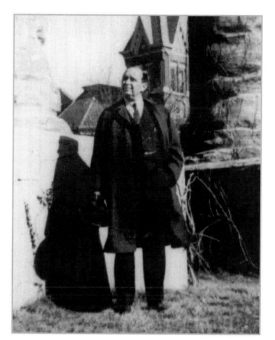

FIGURE 3.74   Dandy visiting his alma mater, the University of Missouri.

REVISITING MISSOURI

For all the years following Walter's graduation from the University of Missouri, he remained very loyal to his alma mater (Figure 3.74).

In 1938, Walter Jr. accompanied his father on a visit to Missouri (Figures 3.75–3.78). They stopped at the University, where Dandy had his picture taken next to the traditional columns. During their stop in Sedalia, young Walter was shown the sights of his father's hometown, including a barn that his father had painted. Remembering his father's tales of its great size, young Walter was amazed at how much it must have shrunk in the intervening years!

The visit in Sedalia with Dandy's old friends is shown in Figure 3.75, below. Present were Polly Battersby Foraker, his childhood friend, her husband, Oliver Foraker, and Polly's widowed mother, Magdalena, who had emigrated with her husband from Barrow in the early 1880s, preceding John Dandy.

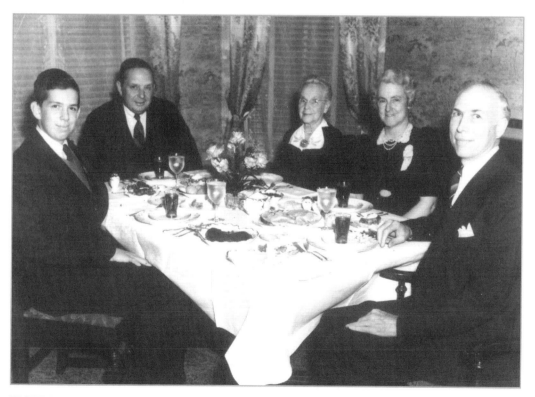

FIGURE 3.75   Walter Sr. and Walter Jr. visiting the Battersby family in Sedalia.

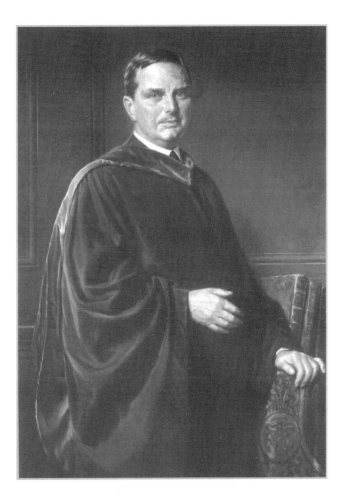

FIGURE 3.76 Portrait of Walter Dandy by Julian Lamar.

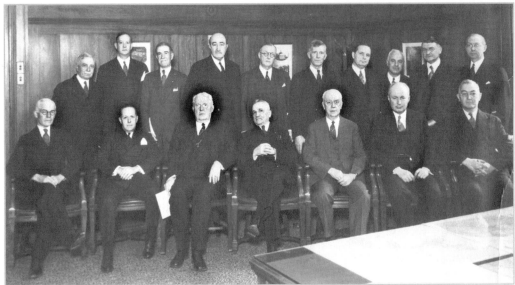

FIGURE 3.77 Walter Dandy on the Board of Overseers, University of Missouri (fourth from the right, second row), 1938.

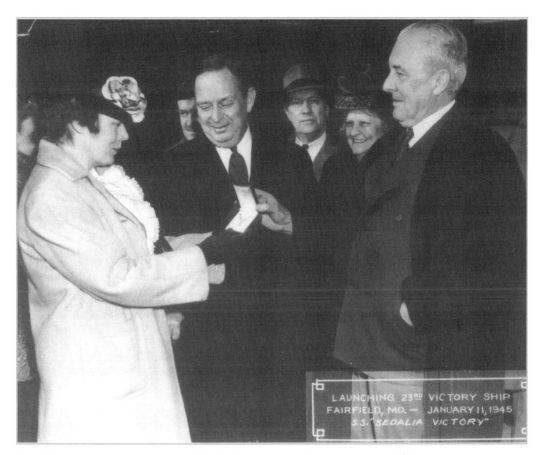

FIGURE 3.78   Christening the SS Sedalia Victory, at the Bethlehem Fairfield Shipyard in Baltimore, during World War II.

Colleagues at Hopkins

One of great benefits of being at Hopkins was the opportunity to work with the other fine doctors whom it attracted (Figures 3.79–3.83). Dandy worked closely with such fine Hopkins professors as pediatrician Ned Park, surgeon Al Blalock, neurologist Frank Ford, and otolaryngologist Ed Broyles, among others, some of whom are pictured here. Many surgeons from other countries visited Hopkins to meet with Dandy, and some came to work with him. Among the thirty-seven foreign "voluntary assistants" to Dandy was Ferdinand Verbeek, a Dutch neurosurgeon who became a friend of the Dandy family.

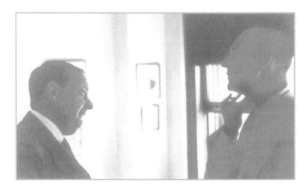

FIGURE 3.79   Dandy in his office consulting with neurologist Frank Ford.

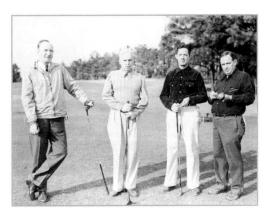

FIGURE 3.80   Ed Broyles, Chalmers Moore, Al Blalock, Walter Dandy.

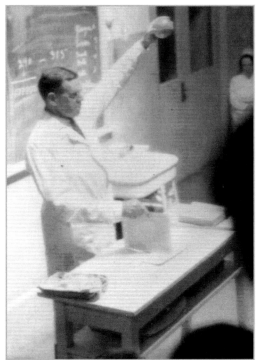

FIGURE 3.81   Pediatrician Ned Park.

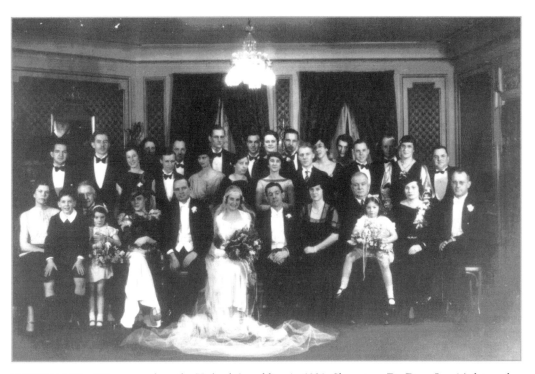

FIGURE 3.82   Kitty remembers the Verbeeks' wedding in 1932. She sat on Dr. Dean Lewis's lap and wore a dress with a butterfly.

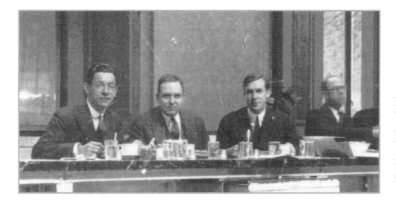

FIGURE 3.83 Ferdinand Verbeek from Holland (left) and Dandy (center). Verbeek was one of many foreign surgeons who studied under Dandy in the 1930s.

Social Life

The Dandy parents' friends were, in general, colleagues from Hopkins (Figures 3.83–3.86). Figure 3.84, below, shows (from the right), Barnes Woodhall and his wife Frances, Dorcas Hager Paget, and the Dandys. Both Dorcas Hager Paget and Frances Woodhall were medical illustrators who studied under master medical illustrator Max Broedel. Dr. Woodhall gave the family their dog, Fagin, an English bull terrier. According to Woodhall, "Mrs. Dandy did become somewhat upset when Dr. Dandy insisted that the dog always sit next to the driver of their auto. Mrs. Dandy or the children had always enjoyed that particular place."[12] Mrs. Woodhall, a member of the 1924 Olympic swimming team, helped teach the Dandy children to swim at Indian Landing on the Severn River.

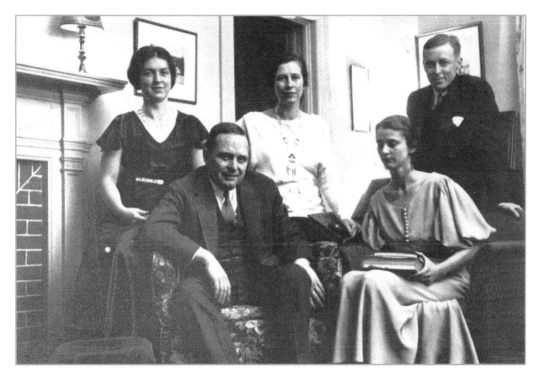

FIGURE 3.84 The Dandys in their living room with Dorcas Hager Padget (center) and Dr. and Mrs. Barnes Woodhall (right).

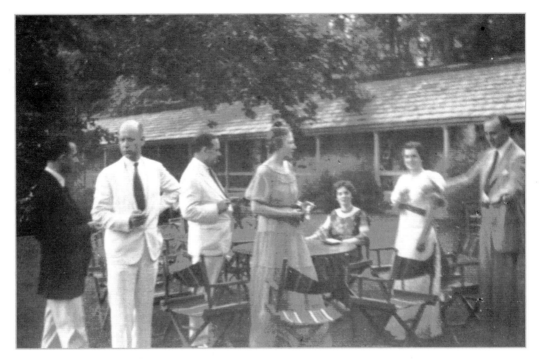

FIGURE 3.85   Friends of the Dandys. From left: Arnold Rich, Frank Ford, Walter Dandy, Mrs. Ford, Mrs. Rich, Sadie Dandy, and Fred Reichert.

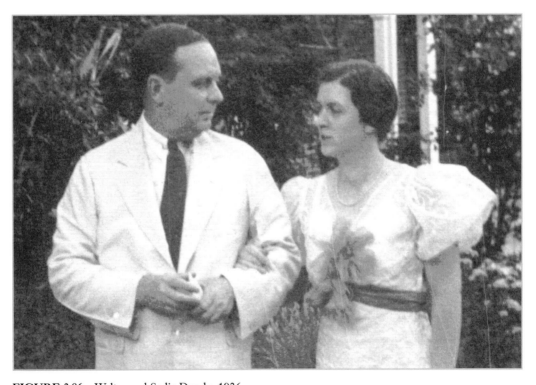

FIGURE 3.86   Walter and Sadie Dandy, 1936.

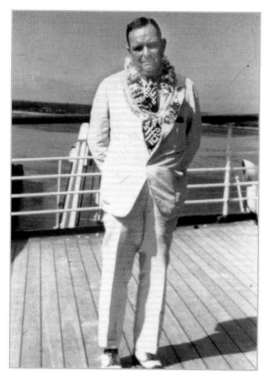

FIGURE 3.87 Dandy on the deck of the Lurline ship as he arrived in Honolulu, 1939.

TRIP TO HAWAII

Walter Dandy loved to travel, but he left the continental United States only a few times after his trip to Europe. He and Sadie drove around the Gaspé Peninsula in Canada in the 1930s, and traveled to Jamaica and the Caribbean on a banana boat later in the '30s. In 1939, Mrs. Dandy was to accompany him to Hawaii to a medical meeting, but young Walter's eye accident kept her home. Dandy, Hopkins colleague Ed Broyles, and Fred Reichert and his family, made the Hawaii trip together.

The Hawaii trip was special (Figures 3.87–3.90). Dandy returned home with Hawaiian shirts, Hawaiian songs on records, and grass hula skirts for his daughters. His father, John, received an enthusiastic letter: "It is probably the loveliest spot on the globe . . . they meet you on the boat with wreaths of flowers. They call them 'lei.' I had six before I reached the Royal Hawaiian Hotel, which is the finest in the world."[13] He and Broyles took a clipper (pontoon aircraft) from Hawaii to San Francisco, much to his delight and probably without Sadie's consent.

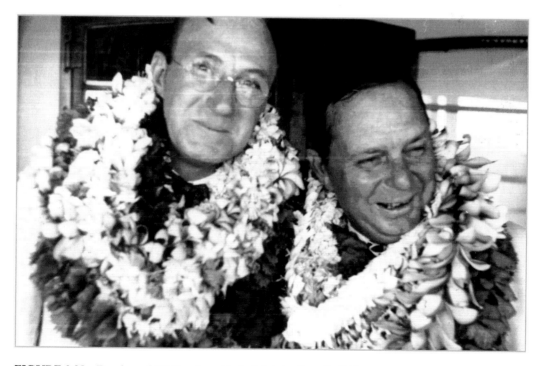

FIGURE 3.88 Dandy and Ed Broyles with their leis in Hawaii, 1939.

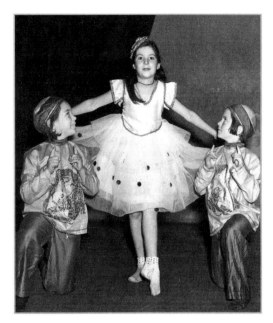

FIGURE 3.89 Kitty (left) and Mary Ellen (right) in a dance recital wearing the outfits their father bought in Chinatown, 1939.

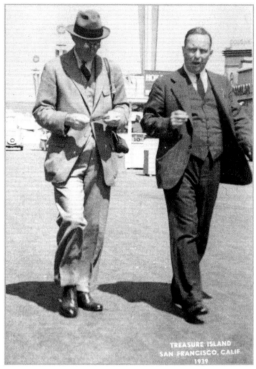

FIGURE 3.90 Dandy and Ed Broyles visiting the World's Fair on Treasure Island in San Francisco Bay, 1939.

Before leaving, he promised Margaret that he would bring her a grass skirt if she stopped sucking her thumb. The bribe worked, but only while he was away. When the grass skirt was securely hers, the thumb came back.

Mary Ellen and Kitty received other surprises-Chinese costumes that he had bought in San Francisco on the way home. In San Francisco, he and Ed Broyles visited Treasure Island, site of the World's Fair.

After the Hawaii trip, the war prevented most travel. Also, Dandy was reluctant to leave his family. Short trips to Ocean City in Maryland and Capon Springs in West Virginia, were sufficient.

TRIPS WITH SADIE TO MEDICAL MEETINGS

Most of Walter and Sadie's trips were planned around medical meetings (Figures 3.91–3.93). They went to a medical meeting in Montana in the early '30s. Figure 3.93 shows the couple in Glacier Park in Montana. Dandy is the "cowboy" on the left.-Sadie is on the big white horse-the one, she said, that always leaned over to eat the thistles on the steep mountain hillside trails! There were many tales of their trip on banana boat in the Caribbean and a stop in Panama.

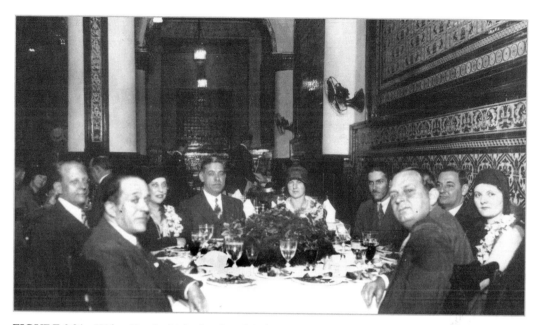

FIGURE 3.91   Walter Dandy (right front) and Sadie Dandy (center) at the Pan Pacific Surgical Meeting in Havana, 1929.

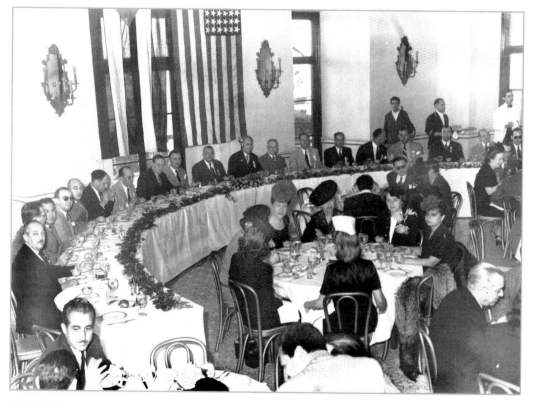

FIGURE 3.92   Dr. Dandy is guest of honor at a medical meeting in Havana. Mrs. Dandy is at the ladies table and is seated at the far end on the right (wearing the smallest hat!), 1945.

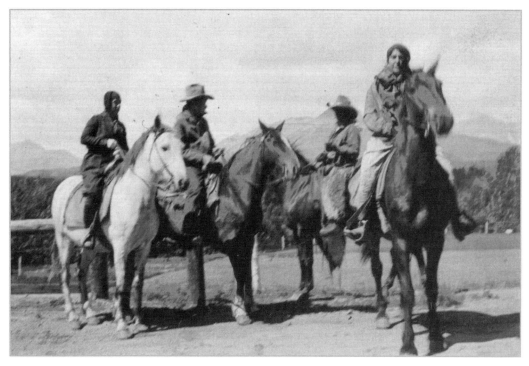

FIGURE 3. 93   Glacier Park in Montana during a medical meeting. Sadie is on the far left, Walter Dandy is the "cowboy" next to her, 1930s.

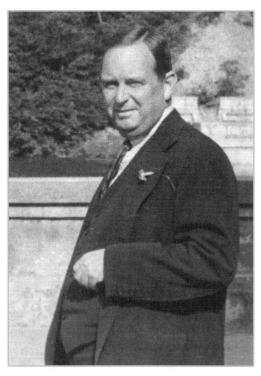

FIGURE 3.94   Dandy as a "Dollar-a-Year Man".

"DOLLAR-A-YEAR MAN"

During the World War I, Dandy had expressed a wish to join the Red Cross ambulance corps so he could see the world. He was kept at Hopkins, however, to fill in for the doctors who had gone to France to serve with the Hopkins Unit.

After the United States entered World War II in 1941, many of his younger colleagues from Hopkins formed the "Hopkins Unit" and served in the South Pacific. In 1942, soon after Pearl Harbor, Dandy offered his services as a civilian consultant to the Navy, "with pay at the rate of $1.00 per annum."[14]

Dandy was pleased to serve his country (Figures 3.94–3.97).

He served under Admiral Ross McIntire, who was also President Roosevelt's personal physician. In his capacity as a "Dollar-a-Year Man," Dandy made an inspection trip of Naval hospitals on the West Coast and Hawaii, accompanied by his fellow neurosurgeon, Captain Winchell ("Wink") Craig, who was on

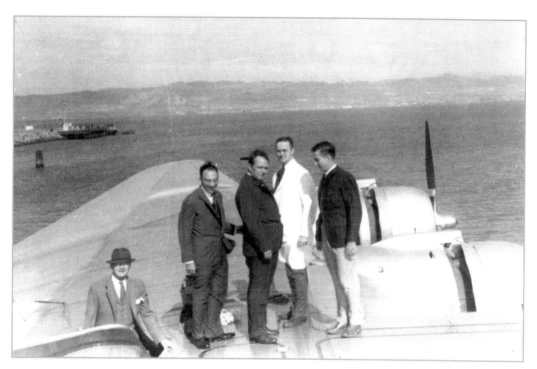

FIGURE 3.95   Dandy at Boeing Field in Seattle.

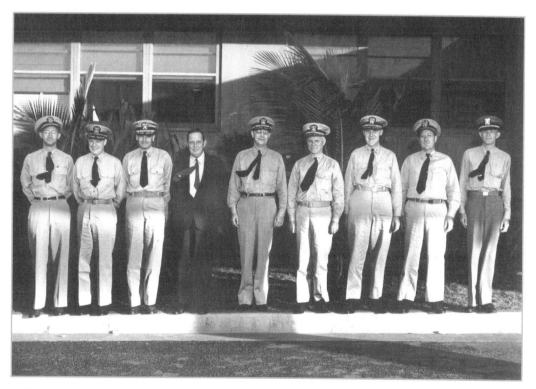

FIGURE 3.96   Dandy (fourth from left), and Navy doctors on tour of inspection, U.S. Navy Pacific Theater. Winchell Craig is on Dandy's left.

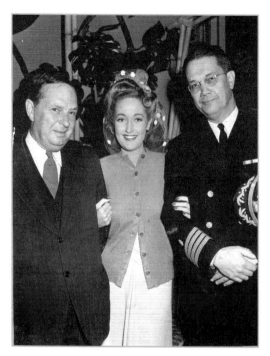

FIGURE 3.97   Dandy, Craig, and Dorothy Lamour.

leave from the Mayo Clinic. In a letter to Sadie he wrote, "Dr. Craig is a fine traveling companion and a real fellow. He knows many more surgeons than I do so he will take me along and I will even up by taking him to see Dorothy! [Lamour, a movie star] He thinks that makes it even!"[15] Dandy had recently operated on Miss Lamour's mother at Hopkins. Dorothy had visited the family and become a friend. He also inspected the hospital at the Great Lakes Training Station in 1943, and found "no weak links in general or in neurosurgery."[16]

CAPON SPRINGS

During the summers of World War II, gasoline rationing had its effect on the family's travel plans. Walter Dandy stayed in Baltimore to work, while the rest of the family (except young Walter, who went to summer camp) drove in the station wagon to Capon Springs in northern West Virginia, and stayed there for most of the summer (Figures 3.98–3.101). Later, Dandy would arrive in his black twelve-cylinder Packard limousine and stay for a few weeks.

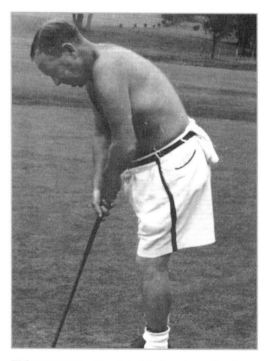

FIGURE 3.98   Dandy in his favorite golf attire at Capon Springs.

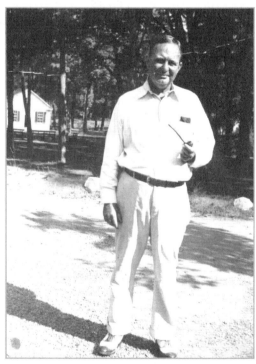

FIGURE 3.99   Dandy enjoying Capon Springs.

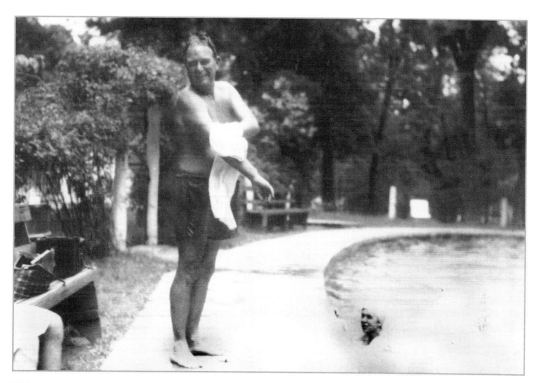

FIGURE 3.100   Dandy after a swim at Capon Springs; Sadie is in the pool (right).

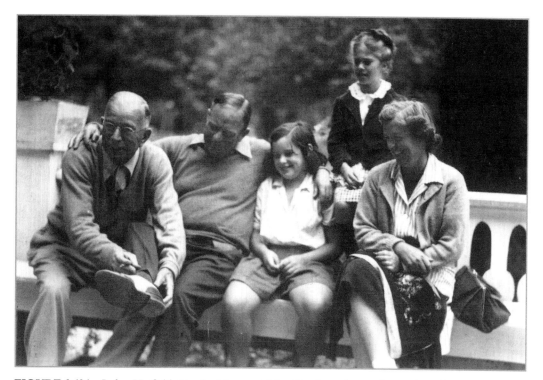

FIGURE 3.101   Judge Hatfield, Dandy, Margaret, Mrs. Dandy and, seated on railing above, Claire Kay Austin enjoying a playful moment.

When Dandy arrived, the pace picked up. His idea of an ideal vacation was eighteen holes of golf, swimming, and then bridge all evening. He vigorously attacked the farm-fresh meals as well. The day began with a before-breakfast swim in the pool, which was cold. His "belly whopper" dive splashed water all over the sides of the pool!

Dandy's usual golf garb (Figure 3.98) was designed to take full advantage of the sun. Even here, his professional services were sometimes needed. Once, when a player on an adjacent fairway was hit in the head with a golf ball, Dandy went over to examine him. The player, not recognizing the professional stature of his casually dressed examiner, said: "I think I will go to Winchester [Virginia] to see a real doctor."

At Capon Springs, Dandy was forced to obey orders from above, something he was not used to doing either at home or at the hospital. Lou Austin, the owner of the resort, always turned the lights out at 11 p.m. and sent everyone home. At first, Walter resisted, telling Austin that he didn't like being treated "like a child." The two eventually worked out their differences and became good friends.

EDUCATION OF THE DANDY CHILDREN

Both Walter and Sadie Dandy stressed the importance of getting a good education. Both parents had skipped a grade and had graduated from high school at age 16. Sadie often reminded the children of their father's excellent grades in school. Much to the children's delight, they found a report card of their father's from grade school. All the grades were excellent, except for deportment! His boyish pranks, including the shaking of the school-room, were noted by the teachers when they graded his behavior.

Walter Dandy was dedicated to providing a good education for his children (Figures 3.102 and 3.103). By the time of Dandy's death in 1946, his son Walter had graduated

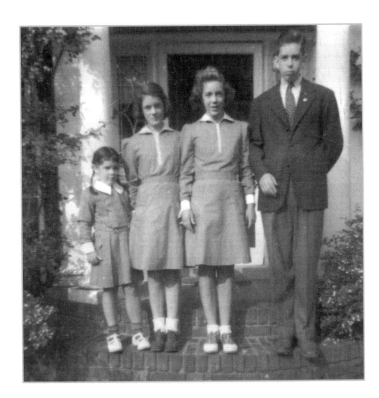

FIGURE 3.102   The Dandy children in 1940.

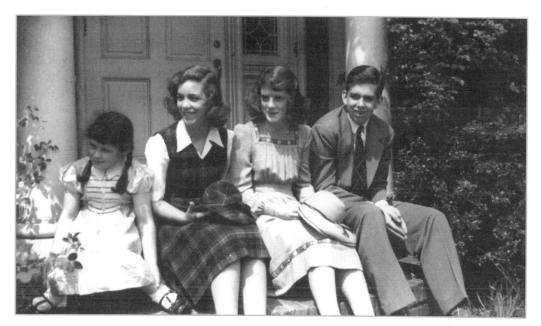

FIGURE 3.103   The Dandy children in their "Sunday Best," 1942.

from Calvert School in 1937, Gilman in 1943, spent 14 months at Princeton and entered the Johns Hopkins School of Medicine in 1944. In 1946, he was a second-year student at the Johns Hopkins School of Medicine.

Mary Ellen had graduated from Calvert in 1939, Roland Park Country School in 1945, and in 1946 was a freshman at Wellesley College.

Kitty had graduated from Calvert in 1940, attended Roland Park for two years, St. Catherine's in Richmond for three years, and had returned to Roland Park in 1945. She was in her senior year there when her father died.

Margaret started at Roland Park, went to Calvert for two years, and was attending Roland Park in 1946.

After Dandy's death, Walter Jr. finished medical school in 1948. Mary Ellen graduated from Wellesley College in 1949, and earned two Master's Degrees in Education: one in General Science and Education from Portland State University in 1970, and one in Health Education from Lewis and Clark College in 1980. Kitty graduated from Wellesley College in 1950. Margaret graduated from Wellesley in 1956 and earned a Master's Degree from the University of Chicago in 1961.

CAREER SUMMARY: "A DEEP VEIN OF TENDERNESS"

In early April 1946, Walter Dandy suffered what was diagnosed as coronary thrombosis. He did not accept the diagnosis, claiming that he was "free from pain" and that it was probably gall bladder colic. But on April 18 he suffered a second heart attack at home. He was rushed to Hopkins where he died the following day, Good Friday, a few weeks after his sixtieth birthday. A service was held at Brown Memorial Presbyterian Church on April 22, conducted by minister T. Guthrie Speers. Walter Dandy was buried in Druid Ridge Cemetery.

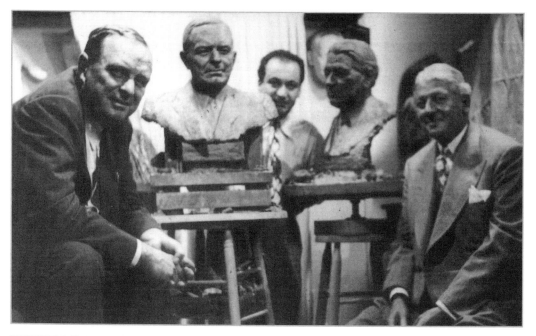

FIGURE 3.104   Dandy and neurosurgeon and amateur sculptor Emil Seletz from Los Angeles.

Dandy had been at Johns Hopkins for thirty-nine years. A prolific surgeon, he is estimated to have performed more than 7,500 surgeries between 1912 and 1946, according
to his biographer.[17]

He published 160 articles, 57 of them in the years from 1930–1939. He also published five complete books and wrote one section in Dr. Dean Lewis's book *Practice of
Surgery.* Two books of his collected writings were published posthumously.

His biographer, William Lloyd Fox, summed up Dandy's career:

> When one looks back on his career of 39 years, several things are apparent. His straight line
> approach to the achievement of superiority in his specialty that reflected both his intellec-
> tual acuity, and power of intense concentration, his constant curiosity about the nervous
> system which he often revealed at surgery by the questions he asked himself aloud How?
> What? Why? Coupled with that curiosity was the courage to break new ground.[18]

An obituary in the *Baltimore Sun* on April 20, 1946, called the readers' attention to
Dandy's human qualities, to a "deep vein of tenderness":

> . . . Dandy contributed other things to the medical school besides his skill and operative
> technique. He contributed a personality that will not soon be forgotten.
>
> After all, Johns Hopkins Medical School is a teaching institution, and Dr. Dandy was a
> remarkable teacher. Gruff of manner, hot of temper, and endowed with a tongue as sharp
> as his instruments, he exacted awe, respect, and the hardest kind of work from his stu-
> dents. They learned the hard way from Dandy but what they earned in the end was all that
> can be learned in the present state of the art. And when they got to know him well, they
> found beneath the hard exterior—as is not uncommon in men of such temperament—a
> deep vein of tenderness. Dr. Dandy lived his professional life among suffering. He could
> exclude the awareness of suffering when this required him to, but he understood it.

$\mathcal{E}$DITORIAL $\mathcal{C}$OMMENT

Marriage, Family, and Career (1923-1946)

By Rafael J. Tamargo, M.D., F.A.C.S., and Henry Brem, M.D., F.A.C.S.

It seems that in 1923, after enduring his rigorous training in general and neurological surgery and probably confident of his promising future at Hopkins, Dandy began to focus on his personal life and growth outside neurosurgery. At the age of 37, not only did he explore life in Europe, but earlier that year became romantically interested in Miss Sadie Estelle Martin. Miss Martin, who had been raised in Baltimore, had graduated from Goucher College in Baltimore in 1921 with a bachelor's degree in nutrition and social science. After a graduate year at the University of Iowa Hospital, she returned to Baltimore to work in the Dietary Department at Hopkins, where she concentrated on diabetic patients. Dandy's first date with Miss Martin was to a football game in Annapolis in October of 1923. They were married at Miss Martin's family home in Baltimore on October 1, 1924, almost a year to the day of their first date.[1] The Dandys had four children: Walter Edward Jr. (born October 1, 1925), Mary Ellen (born July 22, 1927), Kathleen Louise (born August 29, 1928), and Margaret Martin (born January 21, 1935). Dandy considered his family ". . . the finest thing in life."[2]

It is clear from the letters, however, that this incredibly busy man made ample time to be with his wife, four children, and parents, John and Rachel Dandy. Dandy had helped his parents move to Baltimore from Missouri in early 1911, while he worked in a research position under Dr. Harvey Cushing as Assistant in Surgery at the Hunterian Laboratory. Soon after they arrived in Baltimore, Dandy's parents moved again in October 1911 to England and Ireland, where they spent three years. They returned to Baltimore in 1914 after the outbreak of World War I in Europe on July 28, 1914. They then remained in Baltimore close to their only son for the rest of their lives.[3]

Although most neurosurgeons are familiar with Dandy's legendary temper and intensity, few are acquainted with the "deep vein of tenderness" and playfulness evidenced in the letters, recollections, and photographs in the preceding section. His obituary in the *Baltimore Sun* of April 20, 1946, stated:

> . . . Gruff of manner, hot of temper, and endowed with a tongue as sharp as his instruments, he exacted awe, respect, and the hardest kind of work from his students. . . . And when they got to know him well, they found beneath the hard exterior—as is not uncommon in men of such temperament— a deep vein of tenderness. . . .

We see the gentler side of this stern pioneer when he cries at his son's birth and after his mother's death. It is also apparent in his letter to Walter Jr., who was away at camp on the Eastern Shore of Maryland, and whom Dandy attempts to entice back to Baltimore by letting him know how much he and the others miss him. It is also heartwarming that this man who performed so many experiments on dogs obviously had a soft spot for Fagin, his son's English bull terrier, whom he insisted should sit next to the driver in their car, much to his wife's dismay. Incidentally, this dog was a gift from Dr. M. Barnes Woodhall to Walter Jr.[4] Woodhall had been a member of Dandy's brain team and subsequently became a prominent neurosurgeon at Duke University. After Dandy's death Woodhall wrote to Mrs. Dandy that "next to my father, Dr. Dandy did more for me and meant more to me than any other man."[5]

For many years, we have studied Dandy's writings and paused in awe of his surgical and scientific genius. Now, thanks to this book, we become better acquainted with Dandy as a loving and devoted husband, father, and son. As predicted by his obituary, we not only stand in awe of his professional accomplishments, but smile at the tenderness beneath the hard exterior of this great man.

Career: 1923-1946

Although the last 24 years of Dr. Walter Dandy's life (1923-1946) are his peak years of surgical and academic productivity, by 1923 he had already published what some argue are his greatest contributions to neurosurgery: pneumoventriculography and pneumoencephalography. Dandy had graduated from medical school at Johns Hopkins in 1910, at the age of 24, and then finished his residency eight

Continued

years later in 1918, at the age of 32. By 1923, he had established himself as an academic leader in the nascent discipline of neurosurgery by publishing the technique of pneumoventriculography in July of 1918[6] and that of pneumoencephalography in October of 1919,[7] both in the *Annals of Surgery.* The importance of these contributions to neurosurgery cannot be overstated. Whereas pneumoventriculography provided images of the ventricular system after the injection of air into the ventricles, pneumoencephalography provided images of the subarachnoid space after injection of air in the lumbar thecal sac. Therefore, a lesion in the brain, such as a tumor, could be localized by identifying distortions of either the ventricular system or the subarachnoid space. These complementary techniques thus allowed neurosurgeons for the first time to image the silhouette of the brain, localize its pathology, and perform better targeted operations.

Also by 1923, Dandy was already recognized not only as an outstanding academician, but also as a gifted and highly sought-after surgeon. In 1922 he had published another landmark paper in which he described the technique for total resection of cerebello-pontine angle tumors.[8] His surgical skill was widely praised early on in his career. For instance, in early 1918 Dr. Leonard Keene Hirshberg reported in the *New York Sunday American* the operation that Dandy had performed on the son of Harry W. Nice, the future governor of Maryland. The boy had presented with a left upper extremity paresis that resolved after Dandy performed a right craniotomy and removed "six small tumors from the meninges."[9] On January 30, 1919, Abraham Flexner, author of the 1910 Flexner report on American and Canadian medical education[10] and assistant secretary of the General Education Board, wrote to his brother Simon Flexner:

> The general sentiment hereabouts is that Dandy is the man for surgery. ... as Dr. [William Stewart] Halsted comes about very little now, Dandy is carrying the whole thing, and, as far as I can judge, does it admirably. He has the devotion and confidence of all his associates and treats them in a really beautiful way. ...[11]

Given these accomplishments, it is not surprising that by 1921, merely three years after completing his residency, Dandy had received and turned down tempting offers from Baylor University, University of Michigan, Vanderbilt University (chair of surgery), and University of Cincinnati (chair of surgery).[12] Of these, he seriously considered only the position at Cincinnati. After much consideration and a visit to Dr. Halsted in his summer home in High Hampton, North Carolina, Dandy turned down the offer and offered this explanation to Colonel Henry Page, the dean of the University of Cincinnati:

> It was only because I have things here so thoroughly fitted to my needs and desires that I finally found it wiser not to make the change.[13]

It is clear from the preceding section how Dandy had both his professional life at Hopkins and his personal life in Baltimore "thoroughly fitted to [his] needs and desires." Colonel Page then offered the position to another Hopkins surgeon, Dr. George Julius Heuer.[14] Heuer had been three years ahead of Dandy both in medical school at Hopkins and in the Halsted surgical residency. By the time Dandy entered the residency in 1911, Heuer, who had been in neurosurgical training under Cushing since 1907 when he started his internship, was already experienced in neurosurgical procedures. Given that Dandy spent only one clinical year under Cushing (1911-1912), but five years under Heuer (1912-1917), it is possible that Heuer, and not Cushing, had a greater influence on Dandy's neurosurgical training. Indeed, whereas Dandy never co-authored a paper with Cushing, he published three neurosurgical papers with Heuer. Heuer, a forgotten pioneer neurosurgeon of the Johns Hopkins Hospital, went on to an illustrious career in general surgery as chairman of surgery at the University of Cincinnati and then at Cornell University and Dandy stayed at Hopkins as head of the "brain team."[14]

It is with this distinguished background of academic and surgical accomplishments that Dandy sailed for Europe in December of 1923. Apparently, he was encouraged to do so by Halsted and also

Continued

by his friend Dr. Edwards A. Park, who eventually became professor and chief of pediatrics at Hopkins.[15] For this trip, Dandy secured a grant from Flexner's General Education Board of the Rockefeller Foundation[16] and spent four months at the major European cities.[16] From the letters to his parents, it appears that Dandy was more impressed with European culture than with European neurosurgery. Whereas Cushing before him had spent 14 months in Europe (1900-1901) and returned with an expanded neurosurgical horizon,[17] Dandy returned from Europe with the impression that he had not learned much new.[18]

Starting in 1923 and until his death on April 19, 1946, Dandy's surgical and academic productivity was nothing short of prodigious. During these 24 years, he authored 127 articles (out of a career total of 160) and five books.[19] This constituted a publication record of 5.3 articles per year and one book every 4.8 years, which would be considered an impressive output even by today's standards. Furthermore, we must keep in mind that he did this while performing technically complex and often ground-breaking operations four days a week, including Saturdays. During his entire surgical career (1912-1946), Dandy performed at least 7,416 operations,[20] which is an average of at least 212 operations per year, again an impressive performance even by modern standards. A sampling of Dandy's numerous surgical contributions during his last 24 years includes: section of the trigeminal nerve for tic douloureux (1925),[21] total resection of acoustic tumors (1921 and 1925),[8, 22] intervertebral diskectomy (1929),[23] section of the vestibular nerves for Ménière's disease (1933),[24] and resection of ventricular tumors (1933),[25] to mention a few. In addition, in 1938 he reported the first instance of obliteration of an intracranial aneurysm by surgical clipping (which he had performed on March 23, 1937) and thus initiated the modern era of vascular neurosurgery.[26]

Bibliography

1. Fox WL. *Dandy of Johns Hopkins*. Waverly Press, Inc./Williams & Wilkins, Baltimore, 1984, p. 116.

2. Fox. pp. 117, 119, 120.

3. Fox. pp. 29–30.

4. Dandy Jr. WE. Personal communication. 2002.

5. Fox. p. 160.

6. Dandy WE. Ventriculography following the injection of air into the cerebral ventricles. Ann Surg. 68: 5–11, 1918.

7. Dandy WE. Roentgenography of the brain after the injection of air into the spinal canal. Ann Surg. 70: 397–403, 1919.

8. Dandy WE. An operation for the total extirpation of tumors in the cerebello-pontine angle: a preliminary report. Johns Hopkins Hosp Bull. 33: 344–345, 1921.

9. Fox. p. 48.

10. Flexner A. Medical Education in the United States and Canada: A Report to the Carnegie Foundation for the Advancement of Teaching. New York City, Bulletin Number Four, 1910, pp. 346.

11. Fox. p. 54.

12. Fox. pp. 55–56.

13. Fox, p. 56.

14. Borden W, Tamargo RJ. George Julius Heuer, M.D.—Forgotten pioneer neurosurgeon of the Johns Hopkins Hospital. J Neurosurg. June 2002, In press.

Continued

$\mathcal{E}$DITORIAL $\mathcal{C}$OMMENT   *Continued*

15. Fox. p. 85.

16. Dandy-Marmaduke ME. Personal communication. 2002.

17. Fulton JF. Harvey Cushing. A Biography. Charles C. Thomas, Springfield, Illinois, 1946, pp. 161–201.

18. Fox. p. 86.

19. Fox. pp. 261–267.

20. Fox. p. 272.

21. Dandy WE. Section of the sensory root of the trigeminal nerve at the pons. Preliminary report of the operative procedure. Bull Johns Hopkins Hosp. 36: 105–106, 1925.

22. Dandy WE. An operation for the total removal of cerebello-pontine (acoustic) tumors. Surg Gynecol Obstet. 41: 129–148, 1925.

23. Dandy WE. Loose cartilage from the intervertebral disk simulating tumor of the spinal cord. Arch Surg. 19: 660–672, 1929.

24. Dandy WE. Treatment of Meniere's disease by section of only the vestibular portion of the acoustic nerve. Bull Johns Hopkins Hosp. 53; 52–55, 1933.

25. Dandy WE. Benign encapsulated tumors in the lateral ventricles of the brain: diagnosis and treatment. Ann Surg. 98; 841–845, 1933.

26. Dandy WE. Intracranial aneurysm of the carotid artery cured by operation. Ann Surg. 107: 654–659, 1938.

CHAPTER 4

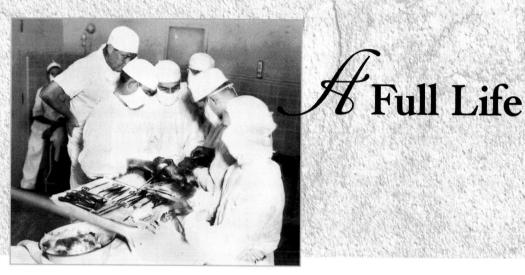

A Full Life

FIGURE 4.1 Dandy observing his colleague, Alfred Blalock.

CHAPTER 4 OUTLINE

- Personality and Style: "A Fortunate Combination of Qualities"
- Dandy the Diagnostician
- Dandy the Surgeon
- Dandy the Teacher
- Dandy the Inventor
- Overview of Walter Dandy's Contributions
- Dandy's Major Contributions to Medicine
- Three Other Contributions to Medicine: Ménière's Disease, Intervertebral Disks, and Patient Care
- Art and Artists
- Famous Patients
- Friends and Relatives of Patients: A Surgeon's Rewards
- Winter Migrations of a Sun Worshiper
- Other Pastimes: Sports, Reading, Writing, Cards, Cars, Trains

PERSONALITY AND STYLE: "A FORTUNATE COMBINATION OF QUALITIES"

Those who worked with Walter Dandy, and even those who lived with him, had conflicting views of what he was really like. Some saw him as an unapproachable professional, others as a warmhearted and generous human being. All recognized that he had definite expectations of what they should be and do, whether the setting was the operating room, the patient's bedside, the baseball stadium, or the home.

Some of his colleagues provide us with astute observations about his personality. One of them, Ned Park, was the professor of pediatrics who had come to Hopkins in 1912 just after Cushing's departure. Park's closeness with Dandy developed as they worked together on sick babies. A month after Dandy's death, Park wrote the following tribute:

> Dandy's relations with other people were unusual. To his friends he was utterly devoted and was unable to see or admit their faults. I recall his devotion to Dr. Dean Lewis [Professor of Surgery at the time] in his final illness; Dandy remained a constant visitor at his bedside until the very end. Dandy was one of the most lovable men I have ever known; he had a most impetuous, warm, affectionate, friendly nature . . . To those whom he did not like he was uncompromising and often he was unable to acknowledge any good in them at all. About people he did not like or respect he was far too open and unrestrained. . . . This was unfortunate, because it created enemies in high places and interfered seriously with the recognition of his accomplishments.[1]

Another colleague, heart surgeon Alfred Blalock (Figure 4.1), also recognized Dandy's warmth, especially in his relationship with his students and associates. Blalock had been a resident at Hopkins in 1928. After some years at Vanderbilt, he returned to Hopkins in 1941 as Chief of Surgery and was Dandy's neighbor and golfing companion. In his memorial tribute, Blalock pointed out that many of Dandy's acts of generosity were not widely known: "The student in need was aided in paying his tuition, the sick house officer or nurse was sent to a resort for a vacation, the orderly was given a home, the surgical department received an anonymous gift. Only the recipients know of these acts of kindness and generosity." Blalock summarized, "Dr. Dandy possessed a fortunate combination of qualities: character, a clear-thinking brain, industry, an intuitive imagination, independence of thought and action, fearlessness and daring, manual dexterity, and a colorful personality."[2]

Although Walter Dandy was known (and feared) for his insistence on high standards of surgical performance, he could be understanding when others on his team made mistakes. Former resident Charles Troland told the story of a resident who had operated on a patient for tic douloureux (trigeminal neuralgia). The operation had been difficult and the patient died. The resident was deeply shaken. That evening, the resident was surprised to receive a call from Mrs. Dandy who asked him to meet Dr. Dandy at the emergency room door. The resident found Dandy there, sitting in his car. Dandy simply waved the resident in to sit beside him for a few moments, then said: "Don't worry, these things happen to all of us."[3]

Dr. Dandy's children were all too familiar with those high standards of performance. When report cards came home with grades that he considered less than the best, he quietly passed the signature requirement on to Sadie. Polished shoes were required-a legacy of William Halsted. Dandy was on the lookout for clean fingernails at dinnertime, especially while the children were digging a hole to China in the lot nearby.

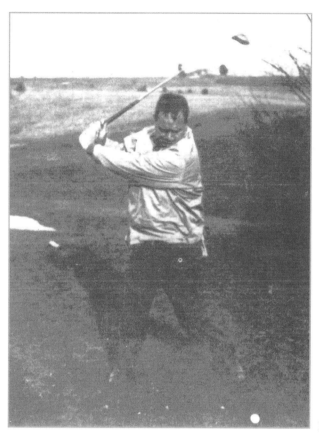

FIGURE 4.2   A "casual" game of golf.

When the high standards of performance in recreational sports were directed to himself, there could be trouble. Figure 4.2 shows Dandy executing what he hoped would be a perfect drive. Golf, like all of Dandy's other activities, was not a casual endeavor. When his golf shot failed to meet his standards, heated words and golf clubs would fly. At Capon Springs, where Kitty often acted as her father's scorekeeper, she would discretely avoid asking for his golf score when a substandard hole was finished. Mary Ellen, embarrassed by her father's outbursts, threatened to stop caddying for him if he continued to throw his clubs and swear. To everyone's great surprise, Dandy restrained himself enough to meet her puritanical requirements, at least while she was his caddy.

Dandy set those high standards aside when he played with his children (Figure 4.3). Dandy's children were impressed by his unmatched skill at spitting prune seeds. Seated on the living room couch, he could spit the seeds across the room into the fireplace. His children were never able to match his skill. He thrilled his children with another game on the same staircase with the beloved sliding banister. The children would sit at the top of the stairs on a runner rug, which he would pull down from the bottom of the staircase. "Here comes the Liberty Limited," he would call out as they thumped their way down to the bottom. Dandy loved to preside over games of "Brother, is you there?" Two children would lie face down on the floor, blindfolded and touching a book set between them with one hand, and wielding a rolled up newspaper in the other. One would call out, "Brother, is you there?" Upon hearing the reply, the first child would take a swipe at the other with

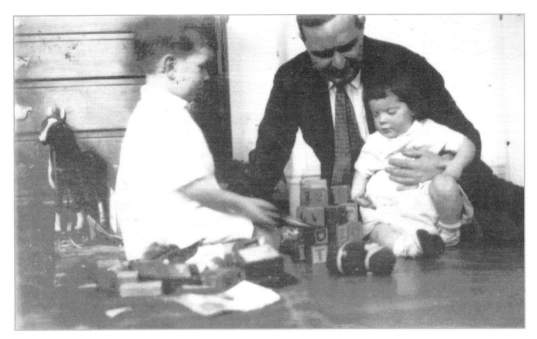

FIGURE 4.3   Playing with Walter and Mary Ellen on the floor.

the rolled up newspaper, and then the roles would be reversed. Sadie would cast a skeptical eye on these raucous games.

Dandy the Diagnostician

Dandy's extraordinary success as a diagnostician was a result of his solid foundation of knowledge he gained this through training and experience, combined with his innate powers of observation. In the early years, he would paste large sheets of paper describing previous cases on the walls of his office. His thirst for knowledge continued throughout his life. Dandy carried on an active correspondence with other neurosurgeons, including those he had first met during his trip to Europe in the 1920s.

Former resident Charles Troland recounted an episode illustrative of Dandy's powers of observation. A patient who had been checked by several physicians had not been given a diagnosis when he came to see Dandy:

> Dandy stood at the foot of the bed and talked to the patient for a few minutes, and then stated that he would take out the tumor the following day. The family and the other doctors were quite upset and finally Dr. Dandy did state that the patient had an acoustic tumor. Dandy added: "Didn't you notice he didn't blink with his left eye?" At surgery the following morning his diagnosis was borne out.[4]

Describing Dandy the diagnostician, Ned Park said, "He seemed . . . suddenly to be seized with intuitions; then almost as if possessed, he would plunge forward with impetuous energy and boldness toward his goal."[5]

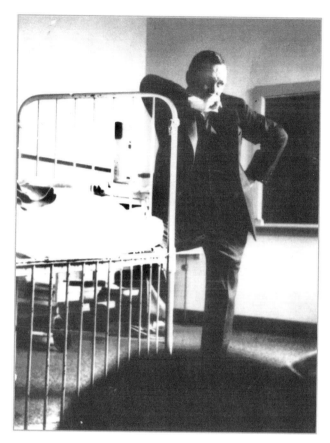

FIGURE 4.4   Dandy concentrating.

Figure 4.4 shows Dandy's intense concentration. Although the photograph has often been reproduced, few people know the circumstances. Barnes Woodhall, who was present when the photograph was taken, wrote many years later: "An unusual feature of this photograph rests in the fact that a student took it with consummate secrecy from the second row of the rounding group."[6] Secrecy was necessary; no distraction would have been tolerated by the "captain" running this tight ship.

DANDY THE SURGEON

Exceptional surgical skill coupled with an indefatigable drive to innovate exemplified Dandy in his role as a surgeon (Figure 4.5). He carried out intricate procedures quickly and with confidence because of his exceptional dexterity which had been honed by extensive practice on animals in the Hunterian Laboratory. Earl Walker, one of Dandy's successors at Hopkins, commended Dandy for his ability "to perform difficult feats of surgery with a relatively low mortality."[7] Peter Jannetta, former Walter Dandy Professor of Neurosurgery at Pittsburgh, has theorized that Dandy must have had excellent eyesight to perform surgeries in which the field was dark and deep.[8]

Dandy's early research into the cause of hydrocephalus and the subsequent development of ventriculography was highly praised by his teacher and mentor, William Halsted,

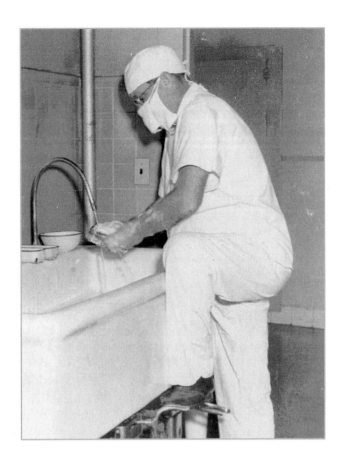

FIGURE 4.5 Scrubbing up before surgery.

in 1918 (see Chapter 2, page 47). A. McGehee Harvey, who became professor of medicine at Hopkins in 1947, wrote in his book *Science at the Bedside,* "Dandy . . . was one of the most imaginative clinical investigators in the history of neurosurgery."[9] Harvey went on to describe Dandy's work on the circulation of cerebrospinal fluid and the cause of hydrocephalus. Harvey observed that, in light of Dandy's talents, "it was but a small step for this genius to conceive injecting air into ventricles thus revolutionizing neurosurgery." (Figure 4.6)

Earl Walker gave special acknowledgment to Dandy's operation for tic douloureux (trigeminal neuralgia), which was easier, simpler and safer than the prevalent technique at the time. In 1995 Donlin Long, a successor of Dandy's at Hopkins, wrote: "Dandy was a surgeon who independently developed a brilliant surgical style not matched before or since, setting technical standards that still excite neurosurgeons."[10]

Barnes Woodhall wrote that the years he worked with Dandy (1927–1935) "were marked by a stream of unusual technical feats of surgery, made possible by accurate localization and Dr. Dandy's unusual courage and skill as a surgeon."[11] Another former resident in the 1940s, Hugo Rizzoli, described Dandy as "a superb and dexterous technician who could be aggressive, radical and innovative when there was hope of effecting a cure for his patient."[12] Fred Reichert, Dandy's first intern, wrote, "In exacting integrity, alert cerebration, and paramount interest in the welfare of each patient, he gave in return a

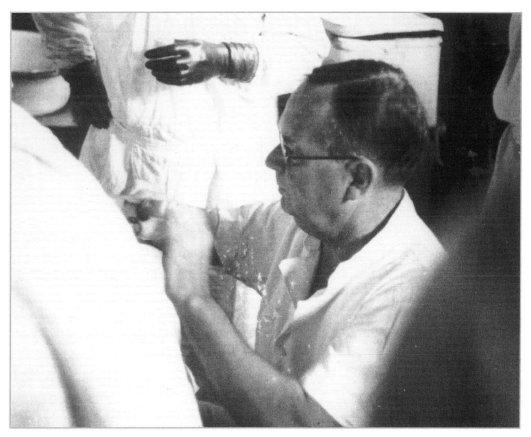

FIGURE 4.6   Performing a spinal tap for a pneumoencephalogram.

share in the diagnostic, operative, and postoperative care of the patient, dependent only upon the ability of his assistant. Not content with existing procedures when these seemed to be inadequate, his keen observation and deduction often led to a solution which meant the saving of a life in an apparently hopeless situation."[13] As Don Long observed, "Dandy was able to develop a philosophy of surgery which is fundamental in neurosurgery today. . . . [He] planned to cure, not palliate."[14] This more extensive surgery involved some element of risk. Dandy had the intellectual independence, skill, and confidence that made innovation possible. As Ned Park put it, Dandy felt "complete skepticism in regard to all accepted ideas."[15]

Don Long was astonished by Dandy's "enormous capacity for work," and cited a figure of 500-700 major operations per year for most of his career.[16] According to Dandy's last resident, Frank Otenasek, even that figure may be too low.

Dandy placed heavy emphasis on patient care. He wrote: "I have always instructed my men [residents] to bear in mind that they must treat patients with the utmost consideration because they need sympathy as well as medical examinations, and this I insist upon. I know that some people are much more difficult to handle than others, but this is a test of their ability as much as a professional test."[17] One of Dandy's innovations was his establishment of a neurosurgical intensive care unit adjacent to the operating room. The unit, which was part of the recovery room, provided improved postoperative care for his patients, and was the first such unit developed.

DANDY THE TEACHER

Dandy's teaching took many forms: formal lectures to medical students, rounds, supervision of surgery of the Brain Team, and lectures to professional organizations around the country. Figure 4.7 shows him lecturing on his method of treating intracranial aneurysms in Atlanta, Georgia. Figures 4.8 and 4.9 show Dandy lecturing in the amphitheater to students. This formal setting was not his preferred style; he was more adept in working with students on rounds. Dandy was most effective as a teacher while he was working with patients; students learned by watching him diagnose and treat his patients (Figure 4.10).

Dandy had a deep respect for teachers because his own teachers had been so important to him, encouraging him throughout his early life. Later, it was his policy not to charge his full fee to teachers.

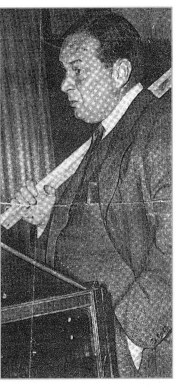

FIGURE 4.7 Lecturing in Atlanta.

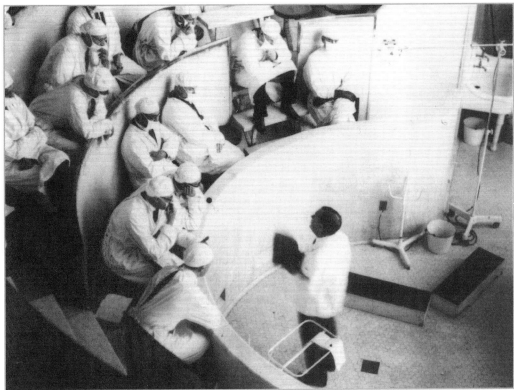

FIGURE 4.8 Dandy teaching in the amphitheater.

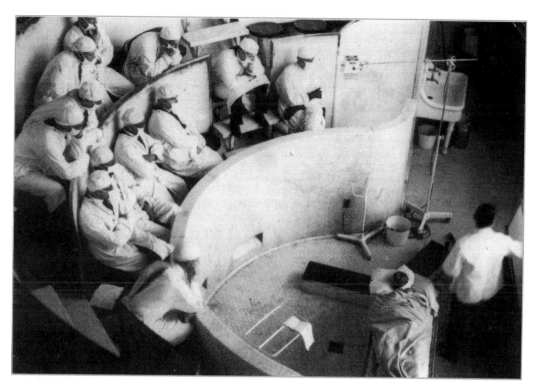

FIGURE 4.9   Dandy teaching in the amphitheater.

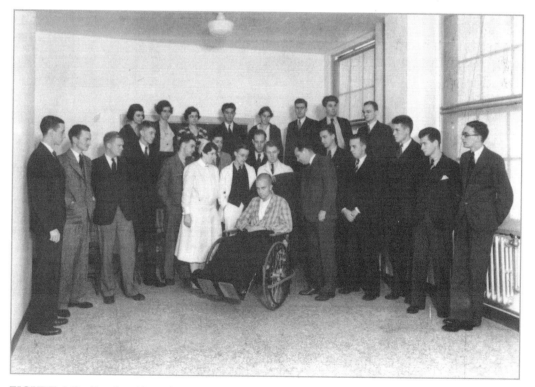

FIGURE 4.10   Dandy with students. (Barner Woodhall is behind the patient to right of the nurse).

DANDY THE INVENTOR

Walter Dandy improved surgical instruments and supportive equipment. In 1927, working with a manufacturer, he designed a special knife "with a long slender handle and a tiny blade at the end for cutting nerves."[18] Dandy developed the ventriculoscope used for cauterization of the choroid plexus in cases of hydrocephalus and a clamp for the edges of the scalp incision now known as the "Dandy Clamp" (Figure 4.11). With assistance from General Electric, he developed a headlight to improve visibility while operating in a darkened room. The contrasting lighting enhanced his ability to discern features in the operating field. When the headlight became available for use in September 1932, Dandy wrote: "It is such a pleasure to work with the new lights, and of course, it means more lives will be saved in this difficult branch of surgery."[19] (See Chapter 3, Figure 3.73, for a picture of this headlight.)

One afternoon in 1940, Brooklyn Dodger player Joe Medwick was "beaned" during a game. The Dodgers' coach Larry McPhail, contacted Dr. George Bennett, an orthopedist at Hopkins, about designing a protective helmet. Bennett referred him to Dandy, who was an avid baseball fan. Dandy had played baseball in his youth and during his years on the house staff at Hopkins. Many of his contemporaries called him "Captain," a vestige of his baseball days. Dandy realized that the protective helmet would need to be simple and easy to wear. He devised the plastic insert shown in Figure 4.12. Developing the prototype of the protective cap became a family project. The children watched their mother spread a sheet of newly developed plastic material on the dining room table, cutting out

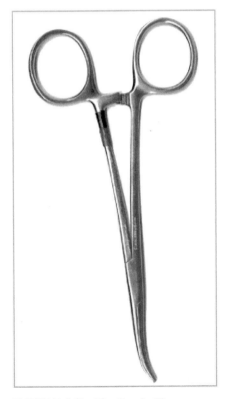

FIGURE 4.11   The Dandy Clamp.

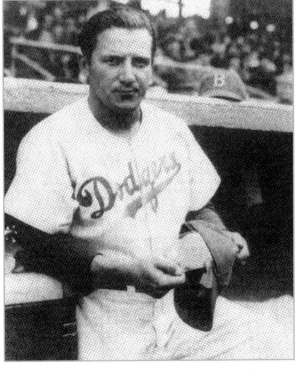

FIGURE 4.12   Joe Medwick of the Brooklyn Dodgers holding the cap, with the plastic insert in his right hand.

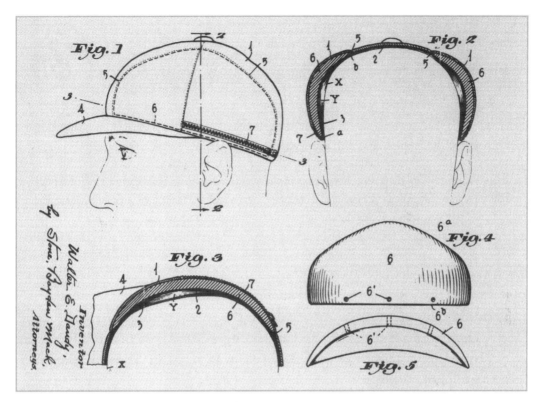

FIGURE 4.13   Drawing of the prototype of the cap.

semicircular pieces and sewing them into a standard baseball cap.[20] The cap was donated to the Baseball Hall of Fame in 1976. The modern fiberglass helmet took its place in 1958.

When Dandy learned that McPhail claimed he had invented the device, Dandy hired a lawyer. In 1943, after a two-year legal contest, the U.S. Patent Office declared Dandy the inventor of the protective baseball cap (Figure 4.13). Dandy had no interest in making money from his invention, but said "I do want the credit for doing something that would be beneficial to baseball."[21]

OVERVIEW OF WALTER DANDY'S CONTRIBUTIONS

Walter Dandy developed a number of innovative surgical strategies that were based on his research on animals and utilized his surgical skill. He also contributed a number of "firsts" to the practice of surgery.

DATE   **DEVELOPMENT**

1912   Discovered the source, flow and resorption of cerebrospinal fluid.

1913   Discovered the cause of hydrocephalus and developed a technique to relieve it.

Continued

1918	Developed ventriculography, which radically improved ability to locate tumors in the brain.
1922	Totally removed acoustic tumors by use of the cerebellopontine angle. This approach was considered "impossible" and "dangerous" because it was beyond the skill level of most neurosurgeons of the day.
1923	Developed the first postoperative intensive care unit next to the operating room for his neurosurgical patients.
1925	Determined the cause of trigeminal neuralgia and used the cerebellopontine angle in its treatment.
1927	Treated glossopharyngeal neuralgia through the head rather than the neck.
1928	Developed the first surgical treatment of Ménière's disease, performing more than 800 operations with only two deaths.
1929	Determined that a ruptured intervertebral disk was the cause of so-called "sciatica" (back pain radiating down the leg) and performed more than 2,000 of these surgeries.

Dandy's Major Contributions to Medicine

Discoveries Related to the Circulation of the Cerebral Spinal Fluid

These three pieces of work made a name for young Dr. Dandy. They are listed together because they are related:

Circulation of the Cerebrospinal Fluid   In 1912, Walter Dandy was given the task of determining the cause of internal hydrocephalus. In the process, he and his colleague, Kenneth Blackfan, determined by insertion of a dye into the ventricle, how the cerebrospinal fluid circulated, as well as where it formed where it and was resorbed. With this information they were able to experiment with animals and were able to produce hydrocephalus in the laboratory.

Hydrocephalus: Cause and Treatment, 1913
Symptoms: Enlargement of the head as a result of abnormal accumulation of cerebrospinal fluid in the brain's ventricular system.

Research: Working on laboratory animals with pediatric resident Kenneth Blackfan, Dandy was able to determine how blockage of the aqueduct of Sylvius could cause hydrocephalus in laboratory animals (Figure 4.14).

Treatment: Dandy developed surgical strategies to treat hydrocephalus in humans (Figure 4.15).

Date: The first paper on hydrocephalus was published in 1913.

This description by Donlin Long reveals a great deal about Dandy as a researcher. As Long describes Dandy's early work on hydrocephalus, Dandy's choice of this topic

> . . . demonstrates one of the keys to Dandy's philosophy. He was willing to choose an extremely difficult subject for study, one with a high risk of failure. Many anatomists and pathologists had failed in their attempts to understand spinal fluid circulation and the genesis of hydrocephalus. Dandy created what many medical historians believe to be the best piece of applied surgical research ever done through technical feats of surgery that none of the pathologic anatomists studying the problem could match. His combination of physiologic and anatomic studies was a masterpiece bringing him instant fame even before he joined the house staff.[22]

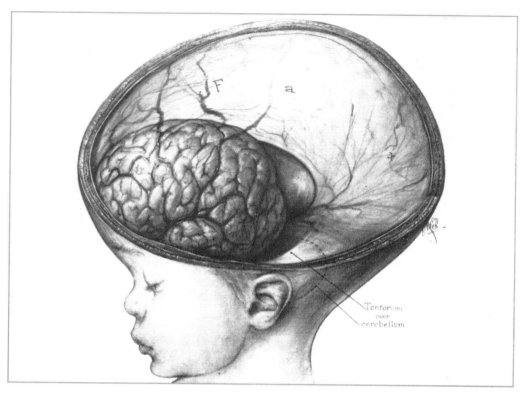

FIGURE 4.14   Illustration showing hydrocephalic baby. (Dorcas Hager, Medical Artist)

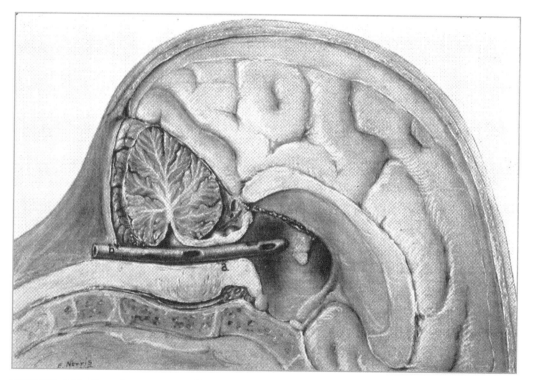

FIGURE 4.15   Stent for treatment of hydrocephalus.

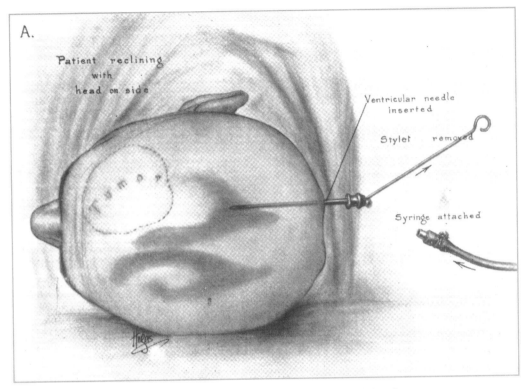

A.

Patient reclining
with
head on side

Ventricular needle
inserted

Stylet removed

Tumor

Syringe attached

FIGURE 4.16 Illustration of ventriculography. (Dorcas Hager, Medical Artist)

From these findings came the development of a new diagnostic technique for clinical use.

Ventriculography and Pneumoencephalography, 1918 Technique: By removing a small amount of cerebrospinal fluid by a lumbar or ventricular puncture, and replacing it with air, the ventricles of the brain can be seen in a clear outline on an x-ray film, since air is less dense than cerebrospinal fluid (Figure 4.16).

Importance: Abnormality of the contour of the ventricle frequently revealed the location of the lesions, which could not be determined by other means. "Dandy found that nearly one-half of all brain tumors are located in the brain stem or cerebellum, where they interfere with the circulation of the cerebrospinal fluid and cause hydrocephalus."[23]

This early work received comments at the time and for years later. Quoting fellow professor William Welch, Halsted wrote to Osler: "Dandy will go far."[24]

Hugo Rizzoli, Dandy's resident in the 1940s, commented:

At the age of 32, Dandy introduced air ventriculography while still a resident. This revolutionized the surgery of the nervous system. Following the advent of ventriculography, accurate localization was possible and Dandy was able to plan the surgical procedures for removing tumors that were never approached before.[25]

Alfred Blalock, M.D., after stating that this was Dandy's greatest contribution, noted that

> At first this method was not received with enthusiasm by most neurosurgeons, but it is used now (1946) in all medical centers and is now regarded by many as the greatest advance ever made in neurosurgery.[26]

This early work made a name for Dandy, not only at Hopkins, but also in the wider medical community. Walter Dandy was nominated for the Nobel Prize for this work.

Innovative Surgical Techniques

Acoustic Tumors   Halsted said that no one makes more than one major contribution to medicine. Walter Dandy proved him wrong: Motivated by the desire to cure, not palliate, Dandy's next discovery was a bold new way to treat acoustic tumors. Previously, Cushing and others had been able only partially to remove tumors of the acoustic nerve, producing palliation but not cure. Dandy was able to accomplish and advocate complete extirpation of these benign brain tumors.

Dandy's work on many types of tumors exemplified his successful pioneering in diverse areas of neurological surgery.[27] But his removal of acoustic tumors was particularly outstanding. Dandy performed the complete extirpation of acoustic neurinomas by the cerebellopontine angle. He published results of twenty-five patients in 1925. He reported on the procedure briefly in the *Bulletin of the Johns Hopkins Hospital* (1929).

The Two Neuralgias: Glossopharyngeal Neuralgia and Trigeminal Neuralgia
Trigeminal neuralgia (TGN) is referred to as "one of the most painful diseases known to man." Glossopharyngeal neuralgia is equally painful. Both types are called tic douloureux.

Trigeminal Neuralgia (Tic Douloureux): 1925[28]
Symptoms: Extreme pain affecting the fifth nerve.
    Previous treatment: Temporal (side) approach.
    Dandy's discovery of the cause of TGN: Dandy was able to determine that this previously idiopathic condition was, in fact, caused in 5 percent of the cases by pressure on the nerve by a tumor in the cerebellopontine angle, and in many others by an artery resting on the sensory root of the nerve (Figure 4.17).
    Dandy's treatment: Using the cerebellopontine approach, as in the acoustic tumors, he was able to partially section the sensory root of the nerve. He felt this approach was superior because it was largely bloodless and it made it easier to preserve the motor root (Figure 4.18).

Glossopharyngeal Neuralgia (Tic Douloureux), 1927
Symptoms: Extreme, spasmodic pain in ninth nerve affecting the tongue, pharynx, and middle ear.
    Previous treatment: Surgical approach through the neck.
    Dandy's treatment: Surgical approach through the cerebellopontine angle, sectioning the nerve. Dandy noted that, to his knowledge, it was the first time this surgery had been performed.[29]

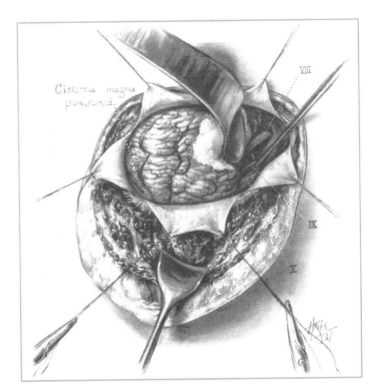

FIGURE 4.17   Surgery for trigeminal neuralgia. (Dorcas Hager, Medical Artist)

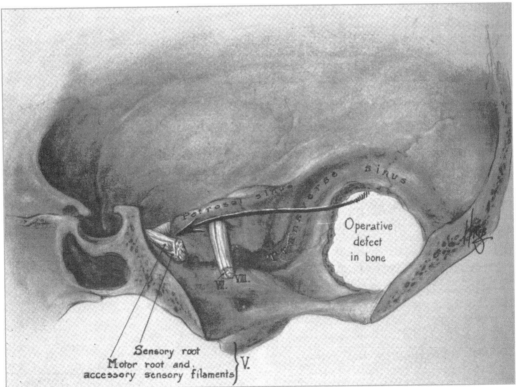

FIGURE 4.18   Illustration of cerebellopontine angle used in trigeminal neuralgia. Note the same approach was used for removal of acoustic tumors. (Dorcas Hager, Medical Artist)

Three Other Contributions to Medicine: Ménière's Disease, Intervertebral Disks, and Patient Care

Ménière's Disease

Symptoms: Severe dizziness, vomiting, and dizziness (Figure 4.19).

Previous treatment: None.

Dandy's surgery: Dandy developed the treatment of Ménière's disease (1928) (Figure 4.20). In this surgery, he sectioned the eighth nerve intracranially. During his career, Dandy performed 692 operations for Ménière's disease with only two deaths, both from infections.[30]

Dandy Cures Malady That Made Luther Throw Inkwell At Satan

Baltimore Brain Specialist Tells Surgeons Of Operation For Relief Of Meniere's Disease

[By the Associated Press]

Philadelphia, Oct. 13—A cure for severe dizziness of a type that caused Martin Luther, the great German religious reformer, to hurl an inkwell at the devil was described today by Dr. Walter E. Dandy, eminent Baltimore nerve specialist.

The Johns Hopkins Hospital brain surgeon told the United States chapter of the International College of Surgeons of an operation for relief of Meniere's disease, an affliction producing such violent dizziness that sufferers occasionally lose their balance and break an arm or leg.

"Luther had it," Dr. Dandy said after his address at the college's second annual assembly. "He threw an inkwell at Satan because the devil was in his ear."

The splotch of ink from a pot tossed by the religious leader can still be seen on the wall of a German schoolroom.

Dr. Dandy said Jonathan Swift, the great English satirist and author of "Gulliver's Travels," also was a victim of the disease. It was called Swift's disease until it was renamed for the French scientist who defined its symptoms.

The dizziness, accompanied by acute nausea and partial deafness in one ear, can be cured by an operation on the eighth cranial nerve, Dr. Dandy said. The surgery involves partial destruction of the nerve, but leaves the hearing fibers intact unless deafness is too far advanced to warrant saving them.

Dr. Dandy said Meniere's disease is "a very common thing—much commoner than is supposed," and can attack anyone. It is not a sequel of other diseases, he said, and is rare in persons under 30. He reported performing 264 operations, the first about ten years ago, without a death.

FIGURE 4.19
Newspaper article from late '20s.

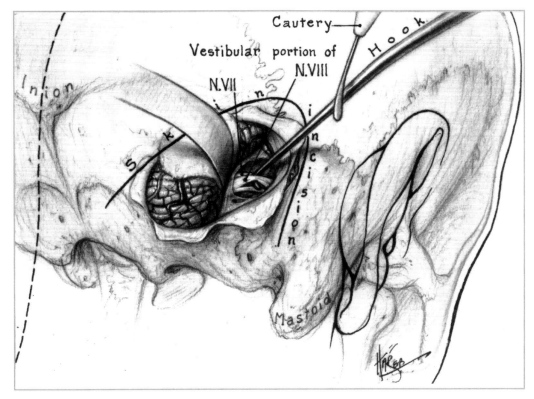

FIGURE 4.20 Surgery for Ménière's Disease. (Dorcas Hager, Medical Artist)

Spinal Surgery

Ruptured intervertebral disk (Figure 4.21).

Symptoms: Pain in lower spine, radiating down one leg, sciatica.

Existing surgery: Dandy's classmate at Missouri and Hopkins, Eustace Semmes, M.D., was performing disk surgeries in the late '30s. Dandy reported on Semmes' surgery as smooth and rapid.

Dandy's surgery: Dandy devised a diagnostic test and operative procedure for the condition.[31] He performed more than 2,000 of these surgeries during his career. Dandy was said to have popularized the surgery.[32]

Patient Care: Recovery Room/Intensive Care Unit

Dandy introduced what may have been the first postoperative recovery room in the history of surgery. He established a three-bed unit, adjacent to the resident call rooms, which was staffed by specially trained nurses day and night. "This was the beginning of careful attention to airway care, temperature control, circulatory monitoring, fluid and electrolyte balance and observation of the state of consciousness of the patient."[33] This intensive care recovery room . . . on the neurosurgical ward . . . unquestionably played a significant role in his low operative mortality."[34]

Note: Walter E. Dandy, Jr., M.D. spent his career as an anesthesiologist at Union Memorial Hospital in Baltimore and was responsible for the intensive care unit at that institution.

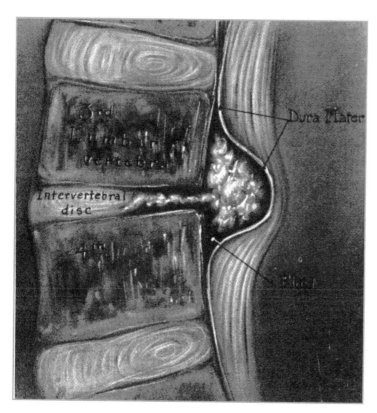

FIGURE 4.21 Illustration of ruptured disk.

Art and Artists

It is no surprise that this astutely observant surgeon was also an accomplished medical artist. His talent as an illustrator was evident in 1906, while still at the University of Missouri, when he drew the detailed drawing entitled "Caput Novum." (See Appendix A.) The article Dandy wrote during medical school article on the smallest embryo in the collection included some of his own illustrations. (See Chapter 2, Figure 2.10.)

During Dandy's medical school years (1907-1910), he had the benefit of instruction by one of the world's foremost medical illustrators, Max Broedel (Figure 4.22). Broedel was a German-trained professor who came to Hopkins in 1894. Broedel coached Dandy as Dandy completed beautiful drawings of the nerve supply and blood supply of the pituitary (See Nerve Supply: Chapter 2, Figure 2.14, Blood Supply: Appendix A.[35])

Broedel's famous etching of William Osler (Figure 4.23) hung in Dandy's Johns Hopkins office in later years. Dandy's children often saw it when they visited. It was magical to Mary Ellen, who thought it depicted Johns Hopkins himself ascending to heaven. The family made an annual visit to visit the Broedels' magnolia tree when it bloomed in the spring, naming it the "strawberry ice cream tree."

In 1926, Broedel's program, Art as Applied to Medicine, attracted Dorcas Hager. She came to Hopkins without any formal training in medical illustration, but chose the Hopkins program to study art and anatomy. She began working with Dandy in 1928 before completing her program in 1929. She became not only an artist, but an anatomist with specialized knowledge of embryology. Although Hager married sur-

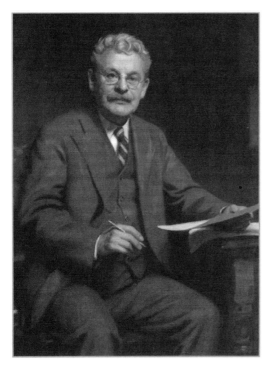

FIGURE 4.22   Max Broedel, medical illustrator.

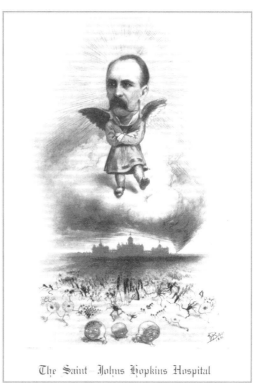

FIGURE 4.23   "Saint Osler," drawing by Max Broedel.

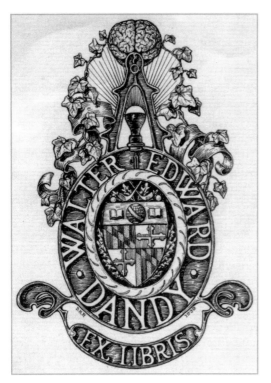

FIGURE 4.24   Walter Dandy's bookplate designed by Dorcas Hager Padget.

geon Paul Padget, she continued to sign her drawings "Dorcas Hager" and Dandy continued to call her "Miss Hager." Dandy had enormous respect for Hager's abilities. At Dandy's urging, she wrote and illustrated "The Circle of Willis: Its Embryology and Anatomy," which Dandy later included in his book *Intracranial Arterial Aneurysms* published in 1944. Dandy also included many of her illustrations in his book *Surgery of the Brain,* published in 1945.

Dandy was especially enthusiastic about the bookplate that Hager designed for him (Figure 4.24). In it, she ingeniously interwove the Hopkins seal, a brain, a pair of rongeurs (plier-like instruments), the ventricles (see lower outer edges of drawing), Dandy's headlamp, and golf clubs. Fox notes: "Despite the occasional clashes of temper between two gifted people, she remained with Dandy until his death."[36]

FAMOUS PATIENTS

Walter Dandy's patients came from all walks of life. One among them was author Thomas Wolfe (Figure 4.25). While in Seattle in 1938, Wolfe developed a severe case of pneumonia, which was followed by intense headaches. An unconscious Wolfe was brought to Dandy in Baltimore by train. Dandy operated, but Wolfe never regained consciousness.[37] He died of tuberculosis of the brain. Wolfe had grown up in Asheville, North Carolina, where his mother ran a boarding house for tuberculosis patients drawn to the town's healthful climate.[38]

Margaret Mitchell (Figure 4.26), author of *Gone with the Wind,* had suffered from back pain for a number of years and came to Hopkins to consult Hopkins internist, Warde Allen. Allen referred her to Dandy. Dandy diagnosed a ruptured intervertebral disk and operated. Later, Mitchell insisted that Dandy had not cured her problem. She complained again and again to him and about him. Dandy told Mitchell that her problem, was, in effect, "all in her head" (a favorite Dandy phrase), and urged her to get back to her work. Needless to say, this infuriated Margaret Mitchell. Despite their common interest in the Civil War, Dandy and Mitchell were never able to resolve their differences. They carried on an extensive and heated correspondence for several years. Forty years later, Sadie Dandy still remembered Margaret Mitchell as having been "a difficult patient."[39]

And then there were the "almost-patients"-those who died before they could be treated. In 1937, Dandy was called to treat George Gershwin for a tumor in the right temporal lobe. He learned at the airport that Gershwin had already died. The circumstances of Gershwin's death were discussed in the *New York Times* in 1998.[40]

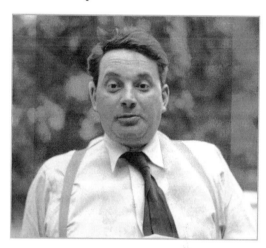

FIGURE 4.25   Thomas Wolfe, Walter Dandy's patient, in 1938.

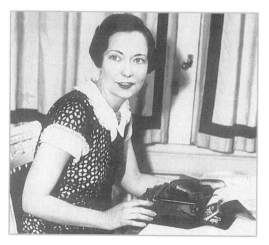

FIGURE 4.26   Margaret Mitchell, author, a patient in 1943.

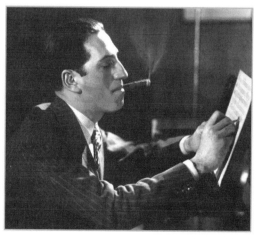

FIGURE 4.27   George Gershwin. (Reprinted with permission of Joanna T. Steichen).

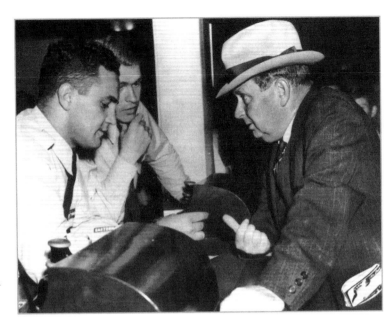

FIGURE 4.28 Walter Dandy at the airport when summoned to treat Trotsky, 1940.

In a similar situation, in 1940, Dandy was called to see Leon Trotsky, the Russian revolutionary, after he was attacked and suffered a brain injury (Figure 4.28). Trotsky died while Dandy was en route.

As mentioned in Chapter 3, page 72, Dandy had another famous patient in the mid-'30s: the Gypsy Queen. There is no mention of her case in the literature, suggesting that others were not as impressed with her status as were the Dandy children.

FRIENDS AND RELATIVES OF PATIENTS: A SURGEON'S REWARDS

Walter Dandy performed many operations for little or no fee, but when the situation allowed, he often charged high fees. Sometimes patients gave him other rewards, including passes to movie theaters, photographs of movie stars, prized objects, and words of praise. These expressions of gratitude meant a great deal to Dandy and his family.

Figure 4.29 is not what it seems. No, Dandy was not summoned to that cheerful bedroom to treat Ronald Reagan. (Reagan can be seen on the bed flanked by Ann Sheridan and Robert Cummings.) Dandy had visited the set of Reagan's movie, *King's Row* as a guest of Emil Seletz, a neurosurgeon and sculptor who was creating a bust of Dandy. Their host was Jack Warner of Warner Brothers Pictures, an old friend of Dandy's, who later gave him a pass to Warner Brothers theaters for the family to use.

One of Ronald Reagan's Hollywood contemporaries was movie star Dorothy Lamour. (Her fabricated name was probably derived from the French word for love, *l'amour,* appropriate to her New Orleans origins.) After Dandy operated on her mother, Mrs. Castleberry (whom he always called Mrs. Cranberry!), Dorothy was a gracious visitor to the Dandy home. In the *Road* movies with Bing Crosby and Bob Hope, she wore relatively little (for the times)-most notably, a South-Seas sarong. The photo (Figure 4.30) was a gift from Lamour for Dandy to hang in his office. She gave each of the children a (less revealing) photograph of herself, as well. The family used the Warner Brothers pass to see the *Road* movies.

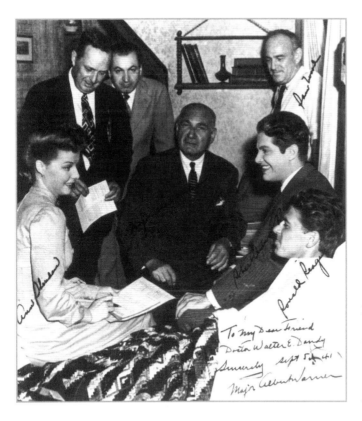

FIGURE 4.29   Walter Dandy (upper left), Emil Seletz, M.D., next to Dandy, Seated: Ann Sheridan, Major Jack Warner, Bob Cummings, and Ronald Reagan on the set of the movie *Kings' Row*, 1944.

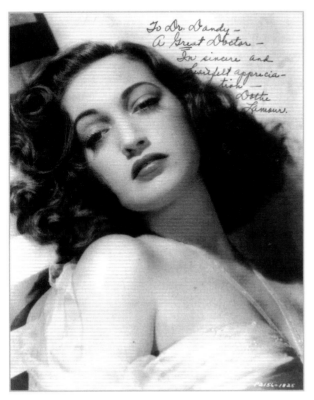

FIGURE 4.30   Dorothy Lamour, 1943.

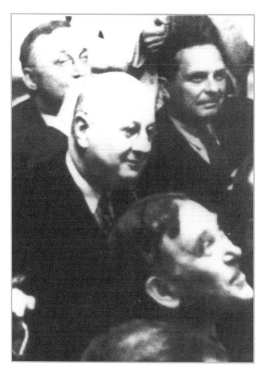

FIGURE 4.31   Walter Dandy (upper right) with Henry L. Mencken, (lower right) at the Pithotomy Club Show, 1938.

Dandy operated without success on the brother-in-law of Richard Kleberg, owner of the enormous King Ranch in Texas. Kleberg's sister expressed her gratitude to Dandy for his treatment of her husband, even though her husband died. After she remarried, she had a son whom she named Dandy Kleberg Johnson. She hosted Walter and Sadie at the King Ranch, an extraordinary experience that they recounted to their children many times afterward.

Henry L. Mencken, the irreverent and acerbic "Bard of Baltimore," was a patient at Hopkins in 1936.

Dear Doctor: My very best thanks for that elegant flask of rye. It undoubtedly saved my life. The brethren have gotten tired of me and so propose to ship me off this afternoon. You were indeed kind to drop in on me and cheer me up. I hope we meet again soon after I escape. Yours, H. L. Mencken

Later, at the time of Thomas Wolfe's hospitalization, Mencken expressed a more earnest tribute to Dandy in a letter to a friend: "The surgeon who attended him is probably the greatest brain surgeon on earth."[41] Mencken appears in the photograph with Dandy attending a 1937 performance at the Pithotomy Club (Figure 4.31), an eating club for students at the Johns Hopkins School of Medicine.

While in Florida in the winter of 1941, Dandy met J. Edgar Hoover, the head of the FBI.[42] Dandy wrote later that he

. . . (had) dinner with him and two of his associates at the Everglades Hotel. I have long admired his work in tracing the kidnappers and other criminals. He is a great fellow and gave me an invitation to bring the kiddies to Washington and see the workings. He was most appreciative of my operation on his man, Lackey [for a] bullet in the spine that Walter saw.[43]

The following winter, the whole family went to Washington, met Hoover, and toured the FBI headquarters. Sadie was most impressed that Hoover had a picture of Shirley Temple on his desk.

WINTER MIGRATIONS OF A SUN WORSHIPER

After Dandy's Jekyll Island experiences from 1916 until 1921, he developed a routine of going south for some time each winter. His first trip after his marriage was to Key West and then to Cuba in 1926. He reported in a letter to his father and mother: "The work has been hard and trying lately . . . and getting away from the rigors of winter . . . I think when I retire, I will just hibernate to Florida."[44]

From Useppa Island, Florida, he wrote: "In my Sedalia days such would have seemed an impossibility. I am very fortunate to be so favored with the superlative type of vacation. . . ."[45] Writing to his parents in 1927, he said

This morning we left . . . at 4 o'clock and fished until 10 and again in the afternoon. It's quite a wonderful sight: about 30 boats running back and forth in a pass about a mile wide. The tides carry you out and you motor back, and do this over and over. I was the first to get a fish, one that weighed 85 pounds. It took 45 minutes to land him. He's as tall as I am. Am having a taxidermist mount him, and some time you will see him over the mantel. The fish leaps in the air several times in the effort to break away. It's a beautiful sight to see him leaping ten feet and assuming a beautiful curve as he goes up and comes down.[46]

This account captures the love of sport that was always part of Walter Dandy's life. The fish also became part of the family's life as an item of household decor after a trip to the taxidermist (Figure 4.32).

While staying at the Boca Raton Club in 1936, he visited a wealthy friend, Mrs. Chadwick, in Palm Beach. Promoting Dandy's business interests, she introduced him to her friends, mostly European nobility. Dandy recounted one of those visits in a letter to Sadie.

A French count is staying at the villa (Mrs. C.) and he wears a monocle and dresses nicely. . . . Social amenities of its proper usage will probably be acquired by an American surgeon before returning to Baltimore. You are missing more than I thought. My practice both foreign and domestic should increase rapidly now, making the trip nice work while in both social and economic ways. Will you stand in my way if I can get a countess? Geist [Dandy's host at Boca Raton and a friend from the Jekyll days] says I should stay here and forget it all. Think what that would mean to my little kiddies to be of great nobility. . . . Love and many kisses to the acme of American nobility.[47]

From Boca Raton, Dandy wrote his parents: "In all my halcyon days, I never saw such finery and luxury. The club roster reads like a directory of Wall Street and big business although not the caliber as old Jekyll [Island] used to show."[48]

During the '40s he stayed at Ponte Vedra in Florida (Figures 4.33).

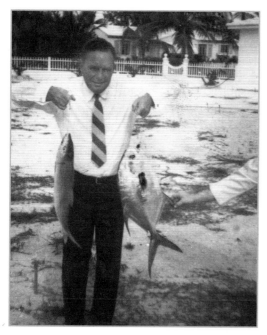

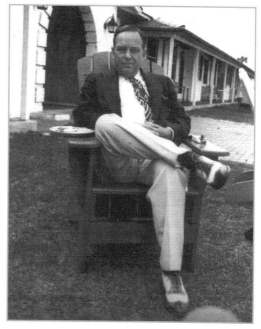

FIGURE 4.32   A day's catch in Florida. This is not *the* tarpon.

FIGURE 4.33   Relaxing at Ponte Vedra, Florida.

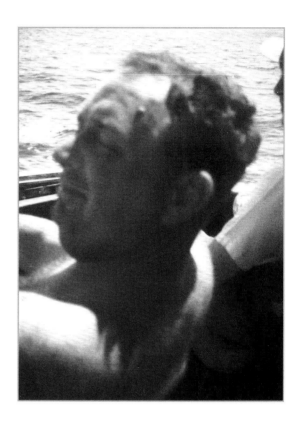

FIGURE 4.34   On a Florida fishing trip in the 1940s.

Other Pastimes: Sports, Reading, Writing, Cards, Cars, Trains

Dandy was an enthusiastic and competitive athlete. He loved to play and to watch others play. He loved baseball, first as a player and then as a fan; he would use his railroad pass on secret trips to watch the New York Yankees. At Hopkins, he learned to play tennis on the courts on the hospital grounds. Sadie used to watch him play before she met him. And there was the golf at Jekyll Island and at home, even Ping-Pong in the cellar. . . . Whatever the sport, he "played to win."[49]

Most of Dandy's reading was nonfiction, with an occasional historical novel. He loved to read about the Civil War, especially a multivolume biography of Robert E. Lee by Douglas Southall Freeman. He liked to tour Civil War battlefields. Walter remembers accompanying his father on a trip to Antietam, planned by Dandy's Hopkins colleague, Ned Park, with Freeman, and Austin Lamont.[50] One of Dandy's treasured possessions was the Matthew Brady photographic series on the Civil War. Dandy's children still remember his pleasure upon opening the package containing the large blue volumes.

Dandy was an avid and tireless bridge player. On Wednesday nights he played with a group of men the Dandy family called "The Bridge Boys." This group included some men who were not physicians, so that if one were called on an emergency, the game did not have to stop. When the group met at the Dandy house, the children were instructed to greet the players and then vanish. The next morning, the living room smelled of smoke, the remains of whiskey, and the favorite snack-which Dandy called "rat cheese"-sharp cheddar. On vacation, he loved to play bridge every night, even after playing golf all day. The family began playing card games with "Go Fish" then progressed to "Hearts" and developed rules that they felt were more interesting than the conventional ones. When alone, Dandy would set up a card table by the living room window and play solitaire. He set up the same table there to do his income taxes, confident that no one he paid could do it better. The children crept around the house, staying out of his way. His disposition deteriorated during the process!

Dandy's love of trains began in Sedalia and continued all his life. At home in Baltimore, he kept a stack of timetables, which he would study during his morning bath. In his early years at Hopkins, he would go to a hillside overlooking the Pennsylvania Station to watch the trains go by. As a consulting surgeon for the Pennsylvania Railroad, he and each of the members of the family were given a pass that allowed them to ride the coach free. Much of Dandy's writing, both letters and articles, was done on the train. He would often use a trip to New York to avoid social obligations. Boarding a Pennsylvania Railroad train, he would settle in a roomette and write all the way to New York and back. During his career, he wrote 160 articles and five books.

Dandy loved cars, and the bigger the better! "Safety considerations" (or so he claimed) were invoked to justify the purchase of an enormous 12-cylinder Packard limousine, complete with fake fur carpeting and folding jump seats. Dandy took advantage of the car's capacity for exceeding the speed limit, as he took advantage of the privileged protection of his physician's plate, a blue cross on a white background, mounted on the front bumper. When he was in a hurry, he could park in the red fire zone with impunity-and, as the children witnessed-sometimes even when there was no emergency.

Walter Dandy: Comments On His Personal And Professional Life

By Edward R. Laws, M.D.

From both a personal and professional standpoint Walter Dandy was certainly a man to be reckoned with. It was my great fortune as a young and developing neurosurgeon to be exposed to numbers of individuals who had intimate professional relationships with Dr. Dandy, and in later years I was privileged to get to know both his wife and his children. During medical school, I was exposed to Dr. Dandy's neurosurgical residents Frank Otenasek and John Chambers, to his nurse anesthetist, Gracie, to a number of general surgeons who had gone through the Halsted training program, having each spent a year on the "Brain Team," and to his colleagues, Dr. Frank Ford in neurology and Dr. Frank Walsh in neuro-ophthalmology. As I stayed on for residency training at Johns Hopkins, I worked directly with doctors Otenasek and Chambers for more than six years. Subsequently, at the Mayo Clinic, my colleague there, Dr. Collin MacCarty, had been a surgical intern assigned to Dr. Dandy; and Dr. MacCarty's wife Margery, as a student and graduate nurse at Johns Hopkins, actually scrubbed for Dr. Dandy in the operating room. Subsequently, in the early years of my career I had a number of "bull sessions" with Drs. Arthur King, Charles Troland, and Barnes Woodhall, all of whom were neurosurgeons who had much of their training with Dr. Dandy. To a man, the neurosurgeons and general surgeons who worked with Dr. Dandy admired and respected him. Most of them called him "the old man" and spoke reverently of his brilliance as a diagnostician and as an innovative surgeon.

Working on the Brain Team must have been close to a religious experience. It was organized in a strictly hierarchical fashion and each member of the team had specific duties and responsibilities down to the intern who was permitted, if talented enough, to pass the instruments at surgery. A typical day started with a morning report to Dr. Dandy as he entered the hospital and walked to the operating room. He would "warm up" with lumbar disc cases and thoracolumbar sympathectomies for hypertension, do some burr holes and inject some air for ventriculography, and then carry on with some posterior fossa operations for trigeminal neuralgia or Ménière's disease and then operate upon a number of brain tumors, after which he would make rounds. For the House Staff, rounds on the neurosurgical service were never actually completed and went on 24 hours a day so that all of the patients could get adequate attention.

Dr. Dandy was an unusual person and had a number of characteristics that allowed him to accomplish so much for neurosurgery. Obviously these same personality characteristics reflected on his family life as well. It is evident that he had a remarkably intact ego that had been carefully nurtured and abetted by his parents. He had a drive for excellence that never ceased and had high standards of personal integrity, self-criticism, and an uncompromising approach to life and work. He was demanding of himself and of others as well. He was a calculated risk taker, an innovator, and had unusual powers of observation with a very "sharp eye" for detail. His intellectual curiosity was at the heart of his ability to make important discoveries in clinical neuroscience. He was intensely loyal to those he admired and dismissive of those he did not, and had a bit of a temper in and out of the operating room. It is curious that he remained relatively aloof from organized medicine throughout his career and was rarely paternalistic with regard to the success and careers of his students. He was able to do large numbers of neurosurgical cases, most of all because he loved surgery, but also because he was extraordinarily well organized and had superb help with the Halsted House Staff as assistants.

Dr. Dandy was a truly genuine person, and he was unsophisticated enough to be forthright in virtually all of his relationships. He was able to enjoy and to take time for recreation and particularly liked playing bridge, fishing, playing golf and traveling. His family represented an important dimension of his life and he was completely devoted to his parents, his wife, and his children.

It is interesting to consider whether Dr. Dandy would have been as successful in his neurosurgical career had he not been exposed to Harvey Cushing. After considerable reflection, I think the answer clearly is that he would, although Dr. Cushing represented both an inspiration and a foil of sorts for Dr. Dandy. What seems to have been critical in the development of Dr. Dandy's passion for neurosurgery was the experience at Johns Hopkins Hospital. The phenomenon of young professors as chiefs of service beginning to develop scientifically based medicine and the whole concept of residency education was undoubtedly a determining factor in Dandy's experience in Baltimore. He learned and applied Halsted's surgical principles and was given a great opportunity to use the laboratory to study a variety of important problems. These included the mechanisms of hydrocephalus, pituitary physiology and metabolism, and ultimately the development of ventriculography and pneumoencephalography.

Like many other great innovators in science, Dr. Dandy's career was a series of accidental and fortunate occurrences. At the University of Missouri he was exposed to scientific mentors who by chance had a relationship with Johns Hopkins School of Medicine. At Johns Hopkins he was filled with the scientifically adventuresome spirit of this new medical school and its new venture in the education of medical and surgical specialists. The accident of Dr. Cushing's departure and the fact that he at the last minute decided not to take Dr. Dandy to Boston with him left Dandy available to fill a residency slot that ultimately became available to him. Although Dr. Heuer took over much of the neurosurgery after Cushing left, when Dr. Heuer departed for a Chair elsewhere, Dandy received his faculty appointment and rapidly matured as a neurosurgical leader.

Many of Dr. Dandy's colleagues felt that his scientific achievements were important enough to warrant consideration of the Nobel Prize in Medicine. A formal nomination was in fact submitted, based primarily on Dr. Dandy's introduction of ventriculography and pneumoencephalography to clinical neuroscience. There is reason to believe that Dr. Dandy might have received this well deserved honor, had it not been for a Swedish member of the Nobel Prize Committee, a neuroradiologist who had played a role in the introduction of air myelography, and effectively blocked the award to Dr. Dandy.

All heroes have some frailties and it is only fair to mention some of these. His temper and his particular kind of summary judgment of individuals and events have already been mentioned. He was a bit hard of hearing and had a terrible memory for individual names, particularly those of patients, residents, and interns. He was a bit overweight and handled his ongoing craving for cigarettes by "borrowing" them from the residents. He was a dogged competitor and, like all of us, he loved to win.

Walter Dandy had a major impact on American Neurosurgery. He combined patient-centered, scientifically-based Neurosurgery with a bold and inquisitive approach to the management of a wide range of neurological disorders.

CHAPTER 5

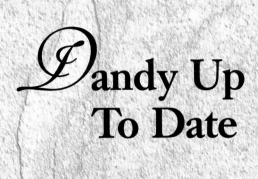

$\mathcal{D}$andy Up
To Date

CHAPTER 5 OUTLINE

LAST WORDS: A POSTHUMOUS ARTICLE

Immediately following Walter Dandy's death, numerous articles and tributes were published, among them the tribute by Dr. Edwards (Ned) Park quoted elsewhere in this book. Park's summary of his friend's contributions to medicine and sensitive insights into his personality appeared in the minutes of the Board of the Johns Hopkins Hospital in May 1946. In August of the same year, the 160th and final article by Dandy, on the center of consciousness, was published posthumously (Figure 5.1).

For a complete list of Dandy's publications, see Appendix. XX. For a list of other tributes and articles about Walter Dandy, see the Bibliography.

WALTER DANDY AS HONORED GUEST OF THE CONGRESS OF NEUROLOGICAL SURGEONS

In 1984, the 34th Annual Meeting of the Congress of Neurological Surgeons (CNS) in New York City honored the memory of Walter Dandy and one of his "former residents," Hugo Rizzoli. Since 1951, the CNS Annual Meeting has featured the contributions of an Honored Guest, but never before had someone been so honored posthumously. The CNS

A—2 * THE SUNDAY STAR, Washington, D. C.
SUNDAY, AUGUST 25, 1946.

Dr. Dandy's Last Paper Locates Brain's Center of Consciousness

By the Associated Press

BALTIMORE, Aug. 24.—The late Dr. Walter E. Dandy, world famous brain surgeon, in a paper published posthumously today in the Johns Hopkins Hospital Bulletin, said he believed he had discovered in which part of the brain the center of consciousness lies.

Dr. Dandy, who died last April, described operations performed by himself and other surgeons over 15 years as supporting a belief that the mysterious entity called consciousness—without which the body becomes a vegetative organism—is fixed in the corpus striatum.

This is a part slightly in front of the mid brain, almost in the center of the skull cavity. It lies on a plane level with the eyes and the top of the ears, about even with the ear tips.

If in its original sense, Dr. Dandy said, consciousness implies the rec- ognition and utilization of incoming impressions, the only way of recognizing consciousness is by the outgoing manifestations of speech and motion.

Dr. Dandy reported on 10 cases involving injury to the front section of the corpus striatum or deprivation of its blood supply. In each case there was complete and immediate loss of consciousness for periods ranging from two to 51 days, followed by death.

During the period of unconsciousness the body was in a vegetative state—all of the automatic functions such as breathing, excretion, operation of the heart and lungs continuing. But there was no sign that the brain was receiving any impressions of the outer world and no response to outer stimuli by speech or movement.

He stated also that the center of consciousness is certainly concerned with sleep.

FIGURE 5.1   Dandy's final article, published posthumously.

President, Edward R. Laws Jr., had so admired Dandy's legacy that he featured him as an Honored Guest for the Annual Meeting that year. Neurological surgeons from around the world attended; the Opening Reception was held aboard the aircraft carrier Enterprise, docked in the New York harbor. Announcement was made of the publication of Walter Dandy's biography, *Dandy of Johns Hopkins*, by William Lloyd Fox, sponsored by the CNS. At the dinner honoring Walter Dandy, his widow, Sadie, spoke briefly. Figure 5.2 shows her presenting a rongeur, one of her late husband's prized surgical instruments, to Dr. Ed Laws.

The Walter Dandy Professorships and Other Honors

In 1985, the Walter Dandy Visiting Professorship was organized at Johns Hopkins Medical Institution, with funds provided by the Dandy family. Each year a visiting neu-

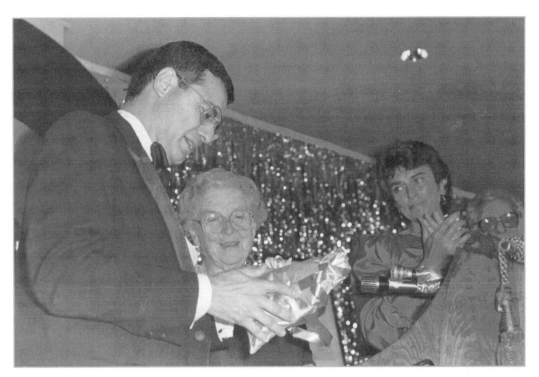

FIGURE 5.2 Mrs. Dandy presenting one of her late husband's surgical tools to Ed Laws, CNS President. Peggy Laws is at right.

roscientist would present a lecture on a topic of current interest, hold seminars and discuss his or her work with Hopkins colleagues, including medical school students. Walter Jr. has been instrumental in the establishment and stewardship of this professorship (Figures 5.3 and 5.4).

In 1986, the University of Missouri Medical School held a meeting "Honoring Dr. Walter Dandy, Class of 1907." At this event, the Walter E. Dandy Neurosurgical Intensive Care Unit was dedicated. Walter Jr. and his mother, then 85, attended the dedication in Columbia, Missouri (Figures 5.5 and 5.6). Other presenters on the program included Ed Laws, Donlin Long, and Hugo Rizzoli, all practicing neurosurgeons whose tributes to Dandy's work appear in this volume. At the meeting, Sadie Dandy returned the academic hood presented to Dandy in 1928. John Oro showed slides of the early photographs of Sedalia and the University, some of which appear in the first section of this album. An article in the local newspaper, the Columbia *Missourian,* quoted Clark Watts, Chief of Neurosurgery at University Hospital, as follows: "Dandy was considered to be a very fatherly man, an excellent teacher, a very concerned surgeon, and an absolutely brilliant innovator. In the first quarter of this century a lot of surgeons were very intense, difficult people but he was not like that at all. He was a gentleman in every sense of the word."[1]

In 1993, the Walter E. Dandy Professorship of Neurological Surgery at the University of Pittsburgh was established by Peter Jannetta, M.D. Dr. Jannetta, an admirer of Dandy's, has refined the surgery for trigeminal neuralgia developed by Dandy in the 1920s. Dr. Jannetta described the process of establishing the professorship, as follows:

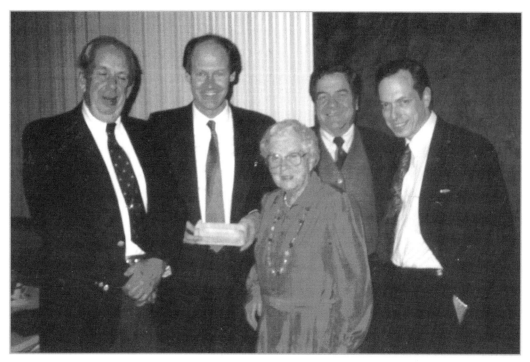

FIGURE 5.3   Walter Dandy, Jr. and his mother, Sadie Dandy, at the 1987 Walter Dandy Visiting Professorship lecture. Show are Walter Dandy, Jr., Thomas Hökfelt (lecturer), Mrs. Dandy, Henry Wagner and Solomon Snyder.

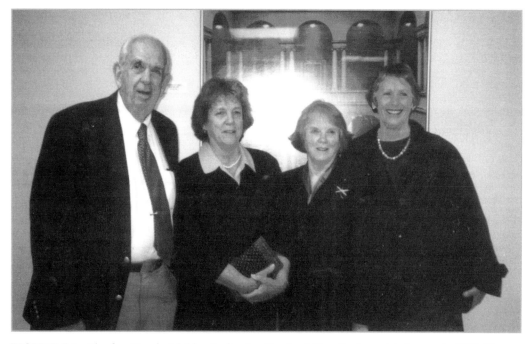

FIGURE 5.4   The four Dandy "children" after the Dandy visiting Professorship lecture in 2000. Show from left: Walter, Jr., Kitty, Mary Ellen and Margaret.

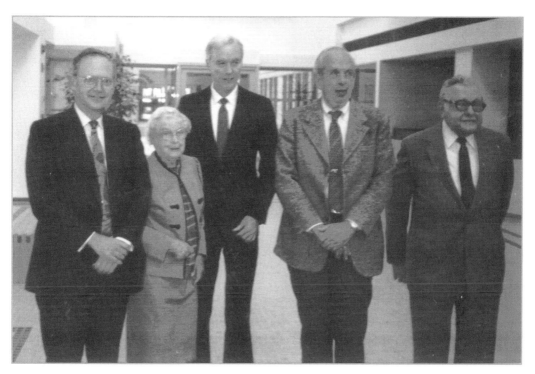

FIGURE 5.5   Sadie Dandy and Walter Dandy, Jr. attend the dedication of the Walter E. Dandy Neurosurgical Intensive Care Unit at the University Hospital in columbia, Missouri, 1986. Also present are Donlin Long (left), Clark Watts (center) and Hugo Rizzoli (right).

Several neurosurgeons of earlier generations have been quoted in my hearing as saying that Walter Dandy saved neurosurgery. There was a time when neurosurgery consisted of a small band of hearty pioneers whose results were not good. As surgeons tried to extend the barriers of ignorance and develop perspectives, procedures and techniques which should help people, they naturally not only helped people but caused side effects. People did not want to go to neurosurgeons. Doctors did not want their patients to go to neurosurgeons. Patients often had late complicated problems where even the best neurosurgeons of today would have had difficulty treating them. The neurosurgeon did not have important ancillary services, studies and colleagues which we expect today. Dandy began the new era of neurosurgery where quality of life rather than just life became important. This has developed magnificently.

I have been asked why we developed a Walter E. Dandy Professorship in Neurological Surgery in Pittsburgh. This came about because it seemed to me in the late 1980s that there should have been one at his institution. We checked with the people at Johns Hopkins and found that there were no plans for such a chair and they were comfortable with us planning one. We were able to use accrued funds and got generous donations from a number of people, including Walter Dandy Jr. to develop a chair which was established in 1993. The current recipient of the chair is Ian F. Pollack, M.D. He is a fitting legatee for the innovative personage that Walter Dandy represented.[2]

Walter E. Dandy, Jr. commented about the event: "This was a remarkable happening, because I know of no other titled chair that was not named for either the donor or the honoree who attracted the funds"[3] (Figures 5.6, 5.7 and 5.8).

As noted in Chapter 4 of this book, Walter Jr. at age 13 had watched his father's operation on Thomas Wolfe in 1938. In the 1990s, Walter Jr. was interviewed by David Herbert

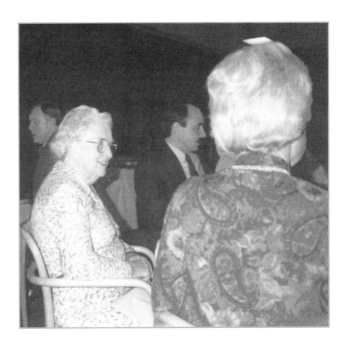

FIGURE 5.6   Mrs. Walter Dandy (left) with John Oro at the dinner following the dedication.

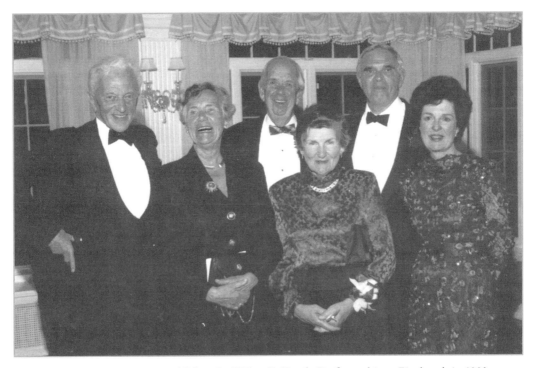

FIGURE 5.7   Peter Jannetta establishes the Walter E. Dandy Professorship at Pittsburgh in 1993. Shown are Peter Safar, Eva Safar, Walter Dandy, Jr., Anne Allen Dandy, Peter Jannetta and Diana Jannetta.

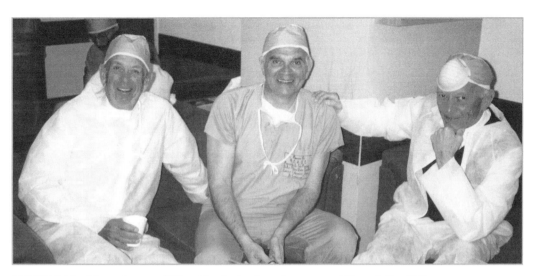

FIGURE 5.8   Three doctors: Walter Dandy, Jr., Peter Jannetta and Peter Safar. 1993.

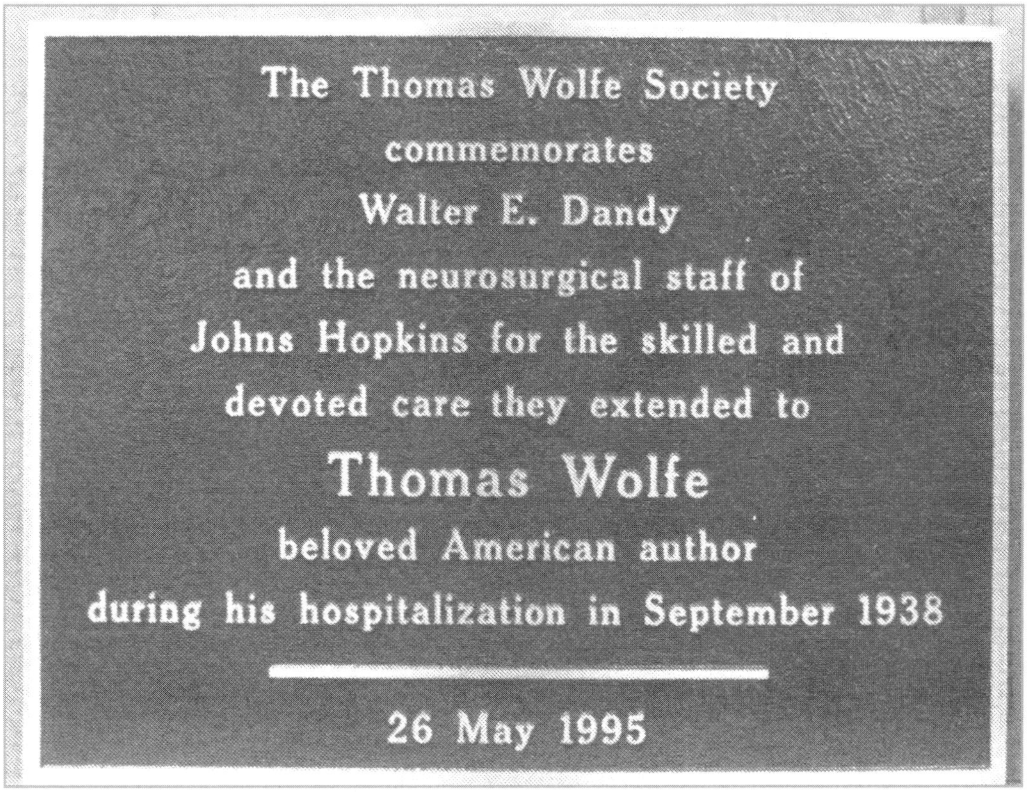

> The Thomas Wolfe Society
> commemorates
> Walter E. Dandy
> and the neurosurgical staff of
> Johns Hopkins for the skilled and
> devoted care they extended to
>
> ## Thomas Wolfe
>
> beloved American author
> during his hospitalization in September 1938
>
> _____
>
> 26 May 1995

FIGURE 5.9   The plaque commemorating Thomas Wolfe's care at John Hopkins Hospital.

Donald, the author of a biography of Wolfe that was published in 1998. In 1995, Walter spoke at the Annual Meeting of the Thomas Wolfe Society at Johns Hopkins, when a plaque about Wolfe's surgery at Hopkins was presented (Figure 5.9) Walter's remarks to the group at that event are set forth in Appendix B.

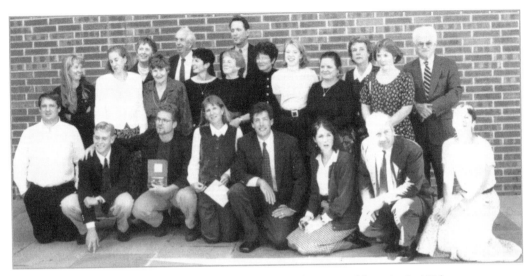

FIGURE 5.10   The Dandy family gathered for Sadie Dandy's memorial service in 1996.

Sadie's Passing and the Preservation of the Dandy Legacy

Walter Dandy died in 1946, at the age of 60. His widow, Sadie, outlived him by fifty years. She never expressed an interest in marrying again, saying that anyone else would be "dull" after Walter. She kept his memory alive for the family until her death at age 95 in 1996. All four of the Dandy children, as well as thirteen of the fourteen grandchildren attended her memorial service in Baltimore (Figure 5.10). It was a memorable event, bringing together family members from all around the country. There are now (in 2002) twenty-four great-grandchildren.

Walter Dandy in the New Millennium

The CNS Walter E. Dandy Orations

In the course of preparations for the golden anniversary of the CNS, the 50th CNS President, Daniel L. Barrow, established the Walter E. Dandy Memorial Oration, a philosophical celebration of Dandy's values and attributes through a lecture by a prominent intellectual on a topic of relevance to humanity at large. This was meant to become the highlight lecture at the Annual CNS Meeting. The First Dandy Oration was delivered by Senator, twice Astronaut and American hero, John Glenn on September 26, 2000, in San Antonio, Texas (Figure 5.12).

The Second Dandy Oration was delivered on October 2, 2001, by famed historian Stephen Ambrose (Figure 5.13) in San Diego, California, at the 51st Annual CNS Meeting presided over by Issam A. Awad, M.D. In his introduction of Dr. Ambrose, Dr. Awad quoted Edward Shil's description of the true intellectual: "In every society . . . there are some persons with an unusual sensitivity to the sacred, an uncommon reflectiveness about the nature of their universe, and the rules which govern their societies."

This characterized Walter Dandy and also the second Dandy Orator Stephen Ambrose. His lecture on the "Essence of Courage and Perseverance" described the role of the American soldier and medic in military epics of the 20th Century. It was particu-

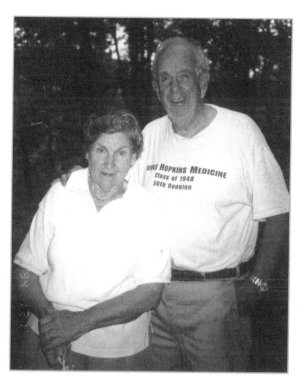

FIGURE 5.11   Walter Dandy, Jr. and his wife, Anne Allen Boyce Dandy, at the 50th reunion of his graduating class at the Johns Hopkins School of Medicine.

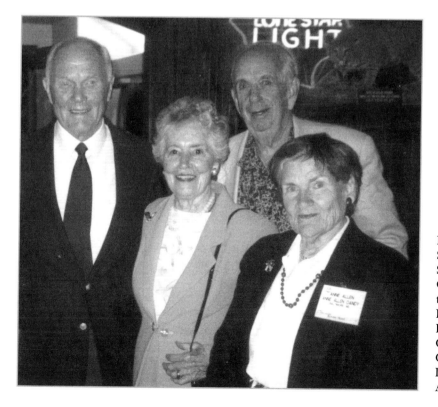

FIGURE 5.12 September 2000: Senator John Glenn delivered the first Walter E. Dandy Oration. From left, John Glenn, Annie Glenn, Walter Dandy, Jr. and Anne Allen Dandy.

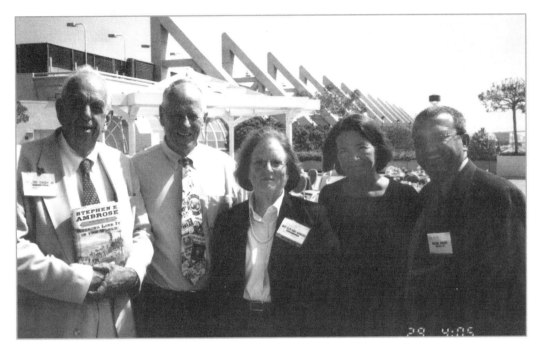

FIGURE 5.13   October 2001, Historian Stephen Ambrose delivered the second Walter E. Dandy Oration. From left, Walter Dandy, Jr., Stephen Ambrose, Mary Ellen Dandy Marmaduke, Moira Ambrose, and Issam Awad, CNS President.

larly timely in light of the tragic events of September 11, only three weeks earlier. The Dandy Oration was a fitting reflection on American leadership in a time of tragedy and challenge.

The Dandy Archives (Website and Information)

Walter Dandy's daughter, Kitty Gladstone, using her earlier career experience as an editor and her lifelong interest in history, looked into the Dandy family history in Tarleton, northwestern England. She interviewed members of the Dandy family (Figure 5.14) including Janet Dandy from Tarleton, England. Janet had written a brief history of her hometown, as well as John Dandy's![4]

Back in this country, Kitty located the correspondence between her father and his parents from 1903-1914 at the Allan Mason Chesney Medical Archives at Hopkins. This extensive correspondence contains more than 200 letters. Kitty edited the letters and many of which are excerpted in this book. A later collection, which includes 125 letters written by Dandy to his family from 1923-1946 were transcribed by Mary Ellen. These letters are excerpted here also.

In a flyer developed by Issam Awad for the CNS Annual Meeting (2001) in San Diego, he wrote:

> Both sets of correspondence (1903-1946) are now available in chronological order with a powerful search engine, posted on the CNS website. These highly personal letters cover Dandy's shy ambition, early career tribulations, rivalry with Cushing, his splendid accomplishments, and the "deep vein of tenderness" so warmly felt by his family. In concert

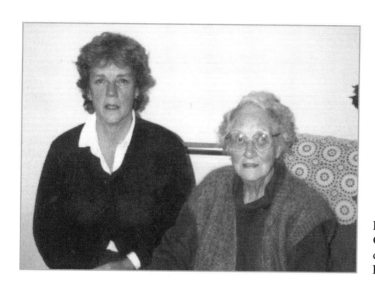

FIGURE 5.14 Kitty Gladstone (left) meets her cousin, Janet Dandy, in England. Mid '90s

with its mission of education, the CNS is grateful to the Dandy family for access to this unique material, and proud to present it to scholars and students of neurological surgery at www.neurosurgery.org/cns/dandy/.[5]

Editorial Comment

Dandy Up To Date: His Legacy in the 21st Century

By Issam A. Awad, M.D.

It is true that neurosurgeons are in love with their history. And they hold a particular passion for the legacy of Walter Dandy. Rising from humble roots in the American Midwest, he defined meritocracy by making a profound impact in the most elite (and elitist) circles of academia and in the emerging field of surgery of the nervous system. He embodied scholarship, surgical virtuosity, and a passion for perfection and innovation. And he was known to tackle the most difficult surgical problems with courage and perseverance, attributes that have become hallmarks of our specialty.

Dandy influenced the field of neurosurgery by helping shape its foundations in the first half of the 20th century. He educated and enlightened colleagues about unique perspectives of neuroanatomy, pathophysiology, and the possibilities and limitations of diagnostic and surgical techniques. And he benefited his own patients and a whole generation of patients treated by other professionals who were so profoundly influenced by Dandy's concepts and ideas. But the true reflection of the meaning and relevance of Dandy's legacy lies in his continued influence during the more than 55 years since his passing. Dandy's values and ideals remain a beacon for the specialty of neurological surgery at the dawn of the 21st century.

Throughout his life, Dandy cultivated a sterling reputation which he earned by helping one patient at a time. And by conquering neurosurgical problems one hill at a time, he championed the neurosurgical contribution as a broader benefit to mankind. Dandy was not a man of the political establishment, but he was respected and revered by those active in neurosurgical politics. His brand of contribution, a caring style of teaching and relentless scholarship, allowed him a prominent place in the halls of academe, even though he was not, by choice, a full-time professor. And the "deep vein of tenderness" so fondly shared with his family and close circle of students, friends, and colleagues, reflects an intensely human side of greatness. Subsequent generations of neurosurgeons have warmly related to Dandy, not only because of the greatness of his scientific and technical accomplishments, but also because of his very human and endearing qualities. Dandy never lost touch with his own humanity and that of ordinary people.

Dandy remained relevant in subsequent generations because of the weight and impact of his contributions. His concepts on hydrocephalus, surgical approaches to inaccessible regions of the brain, and the novel diagnostic and surgical techniques which he revealed and popularized— presented a veritable new body of knowledge characteristic of our specialty. His courage, perseverance, and his unwavering streaks of innovation also defined the epistemology of neurosurgery, and its *modus operandi*. And Dandy's integrity, compassion and his personal warmth, along with an unwavering rigor of standards of excellence, have become the very heart of the ethics and etiquette of our special field. Dandy believed in the breadth, depth, diversity, value and reach of neurosurgery. He seized the small size of our ranks as an opportunity to raise the impact of our contributions.

No wonder Walter Dandy is celebrated so widely by our professional guilds and academic institutions. Named professorships and Dandy orations attempt to convey the special meaning of his legacy to future generations. Dandy remains relevant as the field of neurosurgery enters its second century of contributions. He embodied the neurosurgical ideals, constants among change, through his credibility, compassion, advocacy, scholarship, intellectualism, and not the least, his technical virtuosity. We have already been shaped by the knowledge and techniques that he contributed. Our lives and own contributions can be further enhanced by the influence of Dandy's character and the values he espoused.

End Notes

Chapter ·1

1. The original of this painting was done by Susan Forshaw who lived in Tarleton and was related to the Dandy family. She painted the picture just before the house was torn down. It was copied for the family in 1990.

2. Dandy, John, *My Life History*, 1937. This was handwritten in Baltimore in a small spiral notebook, never published.

3. *Lancashire and Lakeland*, Valentine and Sons, Ltd. London, England (no date). This book was probably purchased by John and Rachel during their visit to England (1911–1914).

4. Dandy, John, letter to Walter, November 15, 1911. Alan Mason Chesney Medical Archives at Johns Hopkins Medical Institutions.

5. Sedalia On Line, http:www.iland,net/sedalia/about (1997).

6. The Kansas line was part of the Union Pacific, Southern Branch.

7. Oro, John, M.D., text and photographs, 1984. Alan Mason Chesney Medical Archives at Johns Hopkins Medical Institutions.

8. Masterson, V. V., *The Katy Railroad and the Last Frontier*, Columbia, Missouri: University of Missouri Press, 1952, p. 255.

9. Dandy, John, letter to Walter, November 15, 1911. Alan Mason Chesney Medical Archives at Johns Hopkins Medical Institutions.

10. Glass, R.L., M.D., "Walter Dandy, Sedalia's Number One Paper Boy," *Missouri Medical*, December, 1965, p. 973.

11. Lang, Hazel, "Shadow of Great Sedalia Scientist Shrinks Little: Dr. Walter E. Dandy, Neurosurgeon, Still Hailed as 'One of the Finest' " *Sedalia Democrat*, 27 June, 1965, Feature Section, p. 1.

12. Dandy, Rachel, England, letter to Walter, c. March 1912, Alan Mason Chesney Medical Archives at Johns Hopkins Institutions.

13. Lang, Hazel, "Shadow of Great Sedalia Scientist Shrinks Little: Dr. Walter E. Dandy, Neurosurgeon, Still Hailed as 'One of the Finest' " *Sedalia Democrat*, 27 June, 1965, Feature Section, p. 1.

14. Lang, Hazel, "Shadow of Great Sedalia Scientist Shrinks Little: Dr. Walter E. Dandy, Neurosurgeon, Still Hailed as 'One of the Finest' " *Sedalia Democrat*, 27 June, 1965, Feature Section, p. 1.

15. Dandy, Walter, letter to his parents, July 30, 1928. Alan Mason Chesney Medical Archives at Johns Hopkins Medical Institutions.

16. Fox, William Lloyd, *Dandy of Johns Hopkins*. Baltimore: Williams & Wilkins, 1984.

16a. "It is remarkable how little insignificant occasions flit through one's mind when passing the scenes of boyhood days. I even thought of how Ervie and I drew a wagon all the way across town to Stevenson's ice plant to bring back ice more cheaply—5¢—and make some salty old ice cream at his house…"

17. www.system.missouri.edu/archives/sigdates.html.

18. Dandy, Walter, letter to his parents, September 7, 1903. Alan Mason Chesney Medical Archives at Johns Hopkins Medical Institutions.

19. Battersby, R.S., letter to Fox, September 1995, quoted by Fox, *Dandy of Johns Hopkins,* p. 12.

20. Lang, Hazel, "Shadow of Great Sedalia Scientist Shrinks Little: Dr. Walter E. Dandy, Neurosurgeon, Still Hailed as 'One of the Finest'" *Sedalia Democrat,* 27 June, 1965, Feature Section, p. 1.

21. Semmes, R.E., M.D., "Walter Dandy, MD, His relationship to the Society of Neurological Surgeons," *Neurosurgery,* Vol. 4, 1979, p. 1.

22. Dandy, Walter, letter to his parents, July 25, 1914. Alan Mason Chesney Medical Archives at Johns Hopkins Medical Institutions.

23. Lang, Hazel, "Shadow of Great Sedalia Scientist Shrinks Little: Dr. Walter E. Dandy, Neurosurgeon, Still Hailed as 'One of the Finest' " *Sedalia Democrat,* 27 June, 1965, Feature Section, p. 1.

24. Fox, p. 18.

25. Osler, William, M.D., letter to Walter E. Dandy, June 25, 1907. Alan Mason Chesney Medical Archives at Johns Hopkins Medical Institutions.

26. Dandy, Walter E., Los Angeles, California, letter to his parents, July 2, 1907. Alan Mason Chesney Medical Archives at Johns Hopkins Medical Institutions.

Chapter 2

1. Johns Hopkins Hospital, "What Hopkins Built and Where," 1997. <http://inot.gdb.org/~pfoster/pa.demo/public_affairs2/basic_facts/hundred>

2. Johns Hopkins Hospital, "What Hopkins Built and Where," 1997. <http://inot.gdb.org/~pfoster pa.demo/public_affairs2/basic_facts/hundred>

3. Johns Hopkins Hospital, "What Hopkins Built and Where," 1997. <http://inot.gdb.org/~pfoster/pa.demo/public_affairs2/basic_facts/hundred>

4. Dandy, Rachel, correspondence, October 30, 1907, Alan Mason Chesney Medical Archives at Johns Hopkins Medical Institutions.

5. Dandy, Rachel, correspondence, December 31, 1907. Alan Mason Chesney Medical Archives at Johns Hopkins Medical Institutions.

6. Fox, William Lloyd, *Dandy of Johns Hopkins*. Baltimore: Williams & Wilkins, 1984, p. 23.

7. Fox, William Lloyd, *Dandy of Johns Hopkins*. Baltimore: Williams & Wilkins, 1984, p. 25.

8. Dandy, Rachel, letter to WED, December 31, 1907. Alan Mason Chesney Medical Archives at Johns Hopkins Medical Institutions.

9. *Neurosurgery*, January 2000 (frontispiece).

10. Harvey, A. McGehee, M.D., Neurosurgical Genius — Walter Edward Dandy, *The Johns Hopkins Medical Journal*, Vol. 135, No. 5, 1974, p. 366.

11. Dandy, Rachel, letter to WED, October 5, 1910. Alan Mason Chesney Medical Archives at Johns Hopkins Medical Institutions.

12. Dandy, John, letter to Hugh Corlett. March 14, 1911. Dandy family collection.

13. Dandy, John, *My Life History* .

14. Blalock, Alfred, M.D., "Walter Edward Dandy 1886-1946," *Surgery*, Vol. 19, No. 5, May 1946, p. 577.

15. Long D. M., M.D., "The Founding Philosophy of Neurosurgery," In Awad, I. A. (ed.), *Philosophy of Neurological Surgery*. Park Ridge, Ill.: American Association of Neurological Surgeons, 1995, p. 3.

16. Crowe, Samuel, M.D., *Halsted of Johns Hopkins: The Man and His Men,* Springfield, Ill.: Charles C Thomas, 1957, p. 86.

17. Crowe, Samuel, M.D., *Halsted of Johns Hopkins: The Man and His Men,* Springfield, Ill.: Charles C Thomas, 1957, p. 86.

18. Flamm, Eugene S., M.D., "New Observations on the Dandy-Cushing Controversy," *Neurosurgery*, Vol. 15, No. 4, October 1994, p. 740.

19. Fox, William Lloyd, *Dandy of Johns Hopkins.* Baltimore: Williams & Wilkins, 1984, p. 67-8.

20. Fox, William Lloyd, "The Cushing-Dandy Controversy." *Surgical Neurology,* Vol. 3, No. 2, Feb 1, 1975, p. 63.

21. Dandy, Rachel, letter to WED, November 6, 1911, Alan Mason Chesney Medical Archives at Johns Hopkins Medical Institutions.

22. Flamm, Eugene S., M.D., "New Observations on the Dandy-Cushing Controversy," (commentary by Edward R. Laws, Jr. M.D.) *Neurosurgery*, Vol. 15, No. 4, October 1994, p. 740.

23. Flamm, Eugene S., M.D., "New Observations on the Dandy-Cushing Controversy," (commentary by Edward R. Laws, Jr. M.D.,) *Neurosurgery*, Vol. 15, No. 4, October 1994, p. 740.

24. Long, D. M., M.D., "The Founding Philosophy of Neurosurgery," In Awad, I. A. (ed.), *Philosophy of Neurological Surgery.* Park Ridge, Ill.: American Association of Neurological Surgeons, 1995, p. 7.

25. Long D. M., M.D., "The Founding Philosophy of Neurosurgery," In Awad, I. A. (ed.), *Philosophy of Neurological Surgery*. Park Ridge, Ill.: American Association of Neurological Surgeons, 1995, p. 8.

26. Dandy, John, letter to WED, November 13, 1911. Alan Mason Chesney Medical Archives at Johns Hopkins Medical Institutions.

27. Dandy, John, letter to WED, November 15, 1911. Alan Mason Chesney Medical Archives at Johns Hopkins Medical Institutions.

28 Dandy, Walter, letter to his parents, August 16, 1914, Alan Mason Chesney Medical Archives at Johns Hopkins Medical Institutions.

29. Dandy, Walter, letter to his parents, October 29, 1914, Alan Mason Chesney Medical Archives at Johns Hopkins Medical Institutions.

30. Sparer, Dot, "Doctoring In Paradise," *Johns Hopkins Medical News*, Winter 2000. p. 18.

31. "Jekyl" was the original spelling. It was changed to "Jekyll" in 1929. The source of this information is Dot Sparer's article.

32. Sparer, Dot, "Doctoring In Paradise," *Johns Hopkins Medical News*, Winter 2000. p. 18.

33. Sparer, Dot, "Doctoring In Paradise," *Johns Hopkins Medical News*, Winter 2000, p. 19.

34. Sparer, Dot, "Doctoring In Paradise," *Johns Hopkins Medical News*, Winter 2000, p. 20.

35. Sparer, Dot, "Doctoring In Paradise," *Johns Hopkins Medical News*, Winter 2000, p. 20.

36. Sparer, Dot, "Doctoring In Paradise," *Johns Hopkins Medical News*, Winter 2000, p. 20.

37. Halsted, William, M.D., Letter to Sir William Osler, 1918, Alan Mason Chesney Medical Archives at Johns Hopkins Medical Institutions.

38. Fox, William Lloyd, *Dandy of Johns Hopkins.* Baltimore: Williams & Wilkins, 1984, p. 69.

39. Walter Dandy, Baltimore, letter to Mrs. Halsted, Letter, Nov. 11, 1922, quoted in Fox, p. 70.

Chapter 3

1. Dandy, Walter E. Letters: December 25, 1923-March 24, 1924. Alan Mason Chesney Medical Archives at Johns Hopkins Medical Institutions.
2. Dandy, Walter E. Letters: 1924-1945. October 1924. Alan Mason Chesney Medical Archives at Johns Hopkins Medical Institutions.
3. Dandy, Walter E. Letters: 1924-1945. October 1924. Alan Mason Chesney Medical Archives at Johns Hopkins Medical Institutions.
4. Fox, William Lloyd, *Dandy of Johns Hopkins.* Baltimore: Williams & Wilkins, 1984, p. 118.
5. Dandy, Walter E. Letters: 1924-1945. June, 1926. Alan Mason Chesney Medical Archives at Johns Hopkins Medical Institutions.
6. Fox, William Lloyd, *Dandy of Johns Hopkins.* Baltimore: Williams & Wilkins, 1984, p. 118.
7. Fox, William Lloyd, *Dandy of Johns Hopkins.* Baltimore: Williams & Wilkins, 1984, p. 142.
8. Fox, William Lloyd, *Dandy of Johns Hopkins.* Baltimore: Williams & Wilkins, 1984, p. 142.
9. Dandy, Walter E. Letters: 1924-1945. July, 1933. Alan Mason Chesney Medical Archives at Johns Hopkins Medical Institutions.
10. Woodhall, Barnes, M.D., "Neurosurgery in the Past: the Dandy Era," *Clinical Neurosurgery,* Vol. 18, No. 1-15, 1971, p. 2.
11. Woodhall, Barnes, M.D., "Neurosurgery in the Past: the Dandy Era," *Clinical Neurosurgery,* Vol. 18, No. 1-15, 1971, p. 7.
12. Woodhall, Barnes, M.D., "Walter Dandy, M.D., personal reminiscences," *Neurosurgery* Vol. 4, No. 3-6, 1979, p. 6.
13. Dandy W.E., Letter to "his father," September 13, 1939. Alan Mason Chesney Medical Archives at Johns Hopkins Medical Institutions.
14. Fox, William Lloyd, *Dandy of Johns Hopkins.* Baltimore: Williams & Wilkins, 1984. p. 207.
15. Dandy, W. E., Letter to Sadie, May 1943. Alan Mason Chesney Medical Archives at Johns Hopkins Medical Institutions.
16. Fox, William Lloyd, *Dandy of Johns Hopkins.* Baltimore: Williams & Wilkins, 1984, p. 208.
17. Fox, William Lloyd, *Dandy of Johns Hopkins.* Baltimore: Williams & Wilkins, 1984, p. 272.
18. Fox, William Lloyd, *Dandy of Johns Hopkins.* Baltimore: Williams & Wilkins, 1984, p. 229.

Chapter 4

1. Park, E.A., M.D., *Walter E. Dandy, M.D. Minute,* Johns Hopkins Hospital, May 6, 1946. Note: The "Minute" tribute is attributed to Park after reading some sections of this article attributed to him in other articles.
2. Blalock, Alfred, M.D. "Walter Edward Dandy 1886-1946," *Surgery,* Vol. 19, No.5, May 1946, p. 577.
3. Fox, J. Dewitt, M.D. "Walter Dandy-Super-Surgeon," *Henry Ford Medical Journal,* Vol. 25, No. 3, 1977, p. 164.
4. Troland, Charles, M.D, Unpublished paper delivered by Troland at the annual meeting of Neurosurgical Society of America, 1965. Quoted by Fox, William Lloyd in *Dandy of Johns Hopkins.* Baltimore: Williams & Wilkins, 1984, p. 154.
5. Park, E.A., M.D., *Walter E. Dandy, M.D. Minute,* Johns Hopkins Hospital. May, 1946.
6. Woodhall, Barnes, "Walter Dandy, M.D., Personal Reminiscences," *Neurosurgery,* Vol. 4, 1979, p. 4.
7. Walker, A. Earl, M.D., "Walter Dandy," *The Founders of Neurology,* 2nd Ed. Springfield, Ill.: Charles C Thomas, 1970, p. 550.

8. Shelton, Mark, *Working in a Very Small Space*, New York: Vintage Books, 1989, p. 45.

9. Harvey, A. McGehee, M.D., *Science at the Bedside*. Baltimore: Johns Hopkins University Press, 1981, p. 76.

10. Long, D.M., M.D., "The Founding Philosophy of Neurosurgery," In Awad, I.A. (ed.), *Philosophy of Neurological Surgery*. Park Ridge, Ill.: American Association of Neurological Surgeons, 1995, p. 7.

11. Woodhall, Barnes, M.D., "Neurosurgery in the Past: The Dandy Era," *Clinical Neurosurgery*, Vol. 18, 1971, p. 6.

12. Rizzoli, Hugo, M.D., "Walter E. Dandy," *Surgical Neurology,* Vol. 2, No. 5, September 1974, p. 294.

13. Reichert, Frederick Lee, M.D., "An Appreciation," *Surgery*, Vol. 19, 1946, p. 580.

14. Long, D.M., M.D., "The Founding Philosophy of Neurosurgery," In Awad, I.A. (ed.), *Philosophy of Neurological Surgery*. Park Ridge, Ill.,: American Association of Neurological Surgeons, 1995, p. 8.

15. Harvey, A. McGehee, M.D. "Neurosurgical Genius-Walter Edward Dandy," *The Johns Hopkins Medical Journal*, Vol. 135, No. 5, November 1974, p. 363.

16. Long, D.M., M.D., "The Founding Philosophy of Neurosurgery," In Awad, I.A. (ed.), *Philosophy of Neurological Surgery*. Park Ridge, Ill.: American Association of Neurological Surgeons, 1995, p. 8

17. Dandy, Walter E., letter to Dr. Caroline Buttrick, Scarsdale, N.Y., November 1, 1937. Quoted in Fox, William Lloyd. *Dandy of Johns Hopkins*. Baltimore: Williams & Wilkins, 1984, p. 164.

18. Fox, William Lloyd. *Dandy of Johns Hopkins*. Baltimore: Williams & Wilkins, 1984, p. 132.

19. Fox, William Lloyd. *Dandy of Johns Hopkins*. Baltimore: Williams & Wilkins, 1984, p. 132.

20. Ledger, Kate, "Capping America's Favorite Pastime," *Johns Hopkins Medical News*, Vol. 20, No. 1, Fall 1996, p. 19.

21. Ledger, Kate, "Capping America's Favorite Pastime," *Johns Hopkins Medical News*, Vol. 20, No. 1, Fall 1996, p. 19.

22. Long, D.M. M.D., "The Founding Philosophy of Neurosurgery," In Awad, I.A. (ed.), *Philosophy of Neurological Surgery*. Park Ridge, Ill.: American Association of Neurological Surgeons, 1995, pp. 7-8.

23. Crowe, Samuel M.D. *Halsted of Johns Hopkins: The Man and His Men*. Springfield, Ill.: Charles C Thomas, 1957. p. 91.

24. Halsted, William, M.D., letter to William Oster, M.D., December 16, 1918, Alan Mason chesney Medical Archives at Johns Hopkins Medical Institutions.

25. Rizzoli, Hugo, M.D., "Dandy's Contributions to the Foundation of Neurological Surgery," *Pediatric Neuroscience*, Vol. 13, 1987, p. 318.

26. Blalock, Alfred, M.D. Walter Edward Dandy 1886-1946, *Surgery*, Vol. 19, No. 5, May 1946, p. 577.

27. Rizzoli, Hugo, M.D., "Walter E. Dandy," *Surgical Neurology*, Vol. 2, No. 5, September 1974, p. 293.

28. Dandy, Walter E. M.D., "Section of the Sensory Nerve at the Pons; Preliminary Report of the Operating Procedure," *Johns Hopkins Hospital Bulletin*, Vol. 36, 1925, p. 106. Quoted by Fox, p. 134.

29. Dandy, Walter E., letter to Ralph Greene, Jacksonville, Florida, April 9, 1927. Quoted in Fox p. 135.

30. Rizzoli, Hugo, M.D. "Walter E. Dandy: An Historical Perspective," *Clinical Neurosurgery*, Vol. 32, Jan. 1, 1965, p. 17.

31. Fox, William Lloyd, *Dandy of Johns Hopkins*. Baltimore: Williams & Wilkins, 1984, p. 150.

32. Crowe, Samuel, M.D. *Halsted of Hopkins, The Man and His Men*. Springfield, Ill.: Charles C Thomas, 1957, p. 103.

33. Harvey, A.M., M.D., *Adventures in Medical Research: A Century of Research at Johns Hopkins*. Baltimore: Johns Hopkins University Press, 1974, p. 65. Quoted in Fox, William Lloyd. *Dandy of Johns Hopkins*. Baltimore: Williams & Wilkins, 1984. p. 83.

34. Rizzoli, Hugo, M.D., "Walter E. Dandy," *Surgical Neurology* Vol. 2, No. 5. p. 294.

35. Fox, William Lloyd. *Dandy of Johns Hopkins*. Baltimore: Williams and Wilkins, 1984, September 1974, p. 30.

36. Fox, William Lloyd. *Dandy of Johns Hopkins*. Baltimore: Williams & Wilkins, 1984, p. 153.

37. Dandy's surgery on Wolfe was observed and later described by Walter Dandy Jr. who was 13 at the time.

38. It is interesting to note that the two articles in the bibliography on Wolfe's surgery were written by Hopkins-trained doctors. Walter E. Dandy Jr. (class of 1948) and S. Robert Lathan (class of 1963). See the Bibliography. See Appendix B.

39. Fox, William Lloyd, *Dandy of Johns Hopkins*, Baltimore: Williams & Wilkins, 1984, p. 188.

40. Carp, Louis, M.D. "George Gershwin-Illustrious American Composer: His Fatal Glioblastoma," *American Journal of Surgical Pathology*, Vol. 3, No. 5, October 1979, pp. 474-478.

41. Brode, Carl. (Ed.) *The New Mencken Letters*, New York: Doubleday, 1977, p. 429.

42. Dandy, Walter E., letter to the family, March 1, 1941. Alan Mason Chesney Medical Archives at Johns Hopkins Medical Institutions.

43. Dandy, Walter E. letter to the family, March 1, 1944. Alan Mason Chesney Medical Archives at Johns Hopkins Medical Institutions.

44. Dandy, Walter E., letter to Mother and Father, 1926. Alan Mason Chesney Medical Archives at Johns Hopkins Medical Institutions.

45. Dandy, Walter E., letter to Sadie and children: May 1928. Alan Mason Chesney Medical Archives at Johns Hopkins Medical Institutions.

46. Dandy, Walter E., letter to Mother and Father, May 17, 1927. Alan Mason Chesney Medical Archives at Johns Hopkins Medical Institutions.

47. Dandy, Walter E., letter to Sadie and children, February 2, 1936. Alan Mason Chesney Medical Archives at Johns Hopkins Medical Institutions.

48. Dandy, Walter E., letter to his parents, January 31, 1936. Alan Mason Chesney Medical Archives at Johns Hopkins Medical Institutions.

49. Fox, William Lloyd, *Dandy of Johns Hopkins*. Baltimore: Williams & Wilkins, 1984, p. 112.

50. Walter commented later that Austin Lamont had "tweaked his interest in anesthesiology." Dandy, Walter E., Jr. *Johns Hopkins Medical School 50th Anniversary Publication*, Baltimore, 1988.

CHAPTER 5

1. Beroset, Deborah, "Neurosurgery Unit to Honor Brains behind Field," *Columbia Missourian*, January 23, 1986. p. A8.

2. Jannetta, Peter, M.D., personal communication to the author, March 14, 2002.

3. Dandy, Walter E. Jr., M.D., *Hopkins Medical News*, Winter 1993, p. 5.

4. Dandy, Janet, *History and Recollections of Tarleton*, Preston, England: Carnegie Press, 1985.

5. Awad, Issam A., M.D. "Flyer about the Dandy Book and Correspondence," Congress of Neurological Surgeons September 2001.

Bibliography: Walter Edward Dandy

Alper, Melvin G. Three Pioneers in the Early History of Neuroradiology: The Snyder Lecture, Documenta Opthalmological 96: 999. pp. 29–49,

Archives of the University of Missouri: //www.system.Missouri.edu/archives/sigdates/html. 02.22.2000.

Baltimore: America's City of Firsts. //www.ci.baltimore.md.us. 1997.

Bercoset, Deborah, Neurosurgery Unit to Honor Brains Behind Field, Columbia Missourian. Thursday, January 23, 1986. p. 8A.

Blalock, Alfred, MD. Walter Edward Dandy 1886–1946. Surgery, May 1946: Vol. 19, No.5, pp. 577–579.

Bliss, Michael. William Osler, A Life in Medicine. Oxford University Press, New York. 1999.

Brem, Henry, MD. In Fundamentals of Surgery, John Niederhuber, Appleton and Lange, a Simon and Shuster Company. 1998. p.733.

Bode, Carl. Ed. The New Mencken Letters, Doubleday, New York. 1977.

Campbell, Eldridge, MD. Walter E. Dandy Surgeon, 1886 –1946. J. Neurosurgery. Vol. VIII, 1951. pp. 249–262.

Carp, Louis, MD. George Gershwin—Illustrious American Composer: His Fatal Glioblastoma. American Journal of Surgical Pathology, Volume 3, Number 5, October 1979. pp. 474–478.

Cooper, I. S., MD. The Vital Probe. Norton, New York. 1981.

Crowe, Samuel MD. Halsted of Johns Hopkins: The Man and His Men. Charles Thomas, Springfield, Illinois, 1957.

Dandy, Janet. History and Recollections of Tarleton. Carnegie Press, Preston, England: 1985.

Dandy, John. Letter to Hugh Corlett. March 14, 1911. Dandy Family Collection

Dandy, Rachel. Letter to Walter and Sadie. December 1924. Dandy Family Collection

Dandy, Sadie M., Letter to John Oro, MD. February 18, 1986 Courtesy or John Oro, MD., University of Missouri School of Medicine.

Dandy, Walter E. A Human Embryo with Seven Pairs of Somites Measuring about 2 mm. in Length, Am. J Anat. 10, 1910. pp. 85–105.

Dandy, Walter E., Correspondence with his Parents: 1903–1911. Edited by Kitty D. Gladstone. 1997. Alan Mason Chesney Medical Archives at Johns Hopkins Medical Institutions, and //www/surgery.org/cns/dandy.

Dandy Walter E. , Letters to his Family: 1923–1946. Edited by Mary Ellen Dandy Marmaduke, 2001. Alan Mason Chesney Medical Archives at Johns Hopkins Medical Institutions, and //www/surgery.org/cns/dandy

Dandy, Walter E. Jr. MD. Thomas Wolfe at Johns Hopkins. Lecture to the Thomas Wolfe Society, Baltimore. 1995.

Dandy, Walter E.,MD. Selected Writings of Walter E. Dandy. Compiled by Charles Troland, MD, and Frank Otenasek, MD. Charles Thomas, Springfield, Illinois. 1957.

Dandy, Walter E., MD. Surgery of the Brain. W.F. Prior Co., Inc., Hagerstown. Md. 1945.

Dr. Walter E. Dandy – One of the World's Greatest Neurosurgeons. BALTIMORE. May, 1946.

Fairman, D. Evolution of Neurosurgery through Walter E. Dandy's Work. Surgery Vol. 19: 1946. pp.583–604.

Flamm, Eugene S., MD. New Observations on the Dandy–Cushing Controversy. Neurosurgery, Vol. 15, No. 4. October 1994. pp.737–739.

Fox, J. Dewitt, MD. Walter Dandy—Super–Surgeon. Henry Ford Hospital Medical Journal. Vol. 25, No.3, 1977. pp. 149–170.

Fox, William Lloyd, PhD. Dandy of Johns Hopkins. Williams and Wilkins, Baltimore, 1984.

Fox, William Lloyd, PhD. The Cushing–Dandy Controversy. Surg. Neurology 3(2).Feb 1, 1975. pp. 61–66.

Fulton, John. Harvey Cushing, A Biography. Charles C. Thomas, Springfield, Illinois. 1946.

Glass, Robert L, MD. Sedalia's Number One Paper Boy. Missouri Medicine. Vol.62. December, 1965. pp. 973–977.

Guitierrez, C. The Birth and Growth of Neuroradiology in the USA. Neuroradiology Vol. 21: 1981. pp. 227–237.

Halsted, William, MD. Letter to Sir William Osler, 1918. Alan Mason Chesney Medical Archives at Johns Hopkins Medical Institutions.

Harvey, A. McGehee, MD. Neurosurgical Genius – Walter Edward Dandy. The Johns Hopkins Medical Journal. Vol. 135, No. 5, November 1974. pp.358–368.

Harvey, A. McGehee, MD. Science at the Bedside. The Johns Hopkins University Press. Baltimore, 1981.

Horowitz, Norman. Library: Historical Perspective of Walter E. Dandy (1886–1946).of Neurosurgery, Vol. 40, No. 3. March, 1997. pp. 646–646.

Jablonski, Edward. George Gershwin: He Couldn't be Saved. New York Times: Letters to the Editor. October 1998.

Jarman, Rufus. Noted Surgeon Here, Reports: Brain Aneurysm Curable. Atlanta Georgian. October 11, 1938.

Johns Hopkins Hospital: What Hopkins Built and Where. http://info.gdb.org/ ~pfoster/pa.demo/ public_affairs2/basic facts/hundred. 1997.

Kevles, Bettyanne. Body Imaging, Newsweek Special Edition. Power of Invention. Winter 1997–1998. pp.74–75.

Kilgore, Erik, J, MD. Walter Dandy and the History of Ventriculography. Radiology 194:1994. pp. 657–660.

Lang, Hazel. Shadow of Great Sedalia Scientist Shrinks Little: Dr. Walter E. Dandy, Neurosurgeon, Still Hailed as "One of the Finest" The Sedalia Democrat, Sunday, June 27, 1965. Feature Section.

Lathan, S. Robert, MD. The Death of Thomas Wolfe: A 60 –Year Retrospective. Journal of the Medical Association of Georgia, September 1998, pp. 214–217.

Laws, Edward, R. Jr., MD. A Neurosurgical Way of Life, 1998 Presidential Address. Journal of Neurosurgery. Volume 89, December 1998. pp. 901–910.

Laws, Edward, R., Jr., MD. Neurosurgery's Man of the Century. The Man and His Legacy. Neurosurgery, vol. 45, no. 5, 1999. pp. 977–982.

Ledger, Kate. Capping America's Favorite Pastime. Johns Hopkins Medical News, Vol. 20, No. 1. .Fall 1996. pp. 18–19.

Ledger, Kate. Safety Did Not Come First. Sports Illustrated, vol 87 (2), July 14. p. 9–10.

Lignon, B. Lee. The Mystery of Angiography and the "Unawarded Nobel Prize: Egas Moniz and Hans Christian Jacobaeus." Neurosurgery, Vol 43, No.3, 1998. pp. 601–611.

Little, John R, MD, Editor, Clinical Neurosurgery, vol.32, Williams and Wilkins, Baltimore, 1984.

Long, Donlin M., MD, PhD, A Century of Change in Neurosurgery at Johns Hopkins, 1889–1989. Journal of Neurosurgery. vol. 71, Nov. 1989. pp. 635–639.

Long, Donlin.M., MD, PhD, The Founding Philosophy of Neurosurgery. In, Awad IA (ed), Philosophy of Neurological Surgery, Park Ridge, Ill., American Association of Neurological Surgeons (Publishers). 1995, pages 1–11.

Masterson, V.V., The Katy Railroad and the Last Frontier, University of Missouri Press, Columbia, Missouri. 1978.

Merrill, J.M. Explanations of Causality, How Margaret Mitchell and Walter Dandy Differed about a Surgical Intervention. Journal of the Medical Association of Georgia. Jul 1: 83(7).1994. pp. 407–408.

Milestones in Medicine. The Hundred Years of the Johns Hopkins Institutions. Sun Magazine May 28, 1989. pp.28–29.

NSYET's Katy Railroads Historical Home Page. http://web2.airmail.net/rvjack. 2/10/97

Park, Edwards A., MD, Walter E. Dandy, M.D. Minute: Adopted by the Medical Board of the Johns Hopkins Hospital, May 6, 1946.

Pinkus, Rosa Lynn, PhD. Innovation in Neurosurgery, Neurosurgery, Vol 4 (5), 1984: pp. 623–630.

Reichert, Frederick. An Appreciation. Surgery Vol. 19, 1946: p. 580.

Rizzoli, Hugo. Dandy's Brain Team. Clinical Neurosurgery Vol. 32. 1985. pp. 23–37.

Rizzoli, Hugo. Dandy's Contributions to the Foundation of Neurological Surgery. Pediatric Neurosci: 13:(6) 1987. pp. 316–322.

Rizzoli, Hugo. Walter E. Dandy, An Historical Perspective. Clinical Neurosurgery 32: Jan 1, 1985. pp. 3–22.

Rizzoli, Hugo. Walter E. Dandy 1886–1946. Surgical Neurology. Vol. 2, No. 5. September 1974. pp. 293–294.

Sachs, E. The Most Important Steps in the Development of Neurological Surgery. Yale Journal of Biology and Medicine Vol. 28. Dec–Feb 1955/6. pp. 444–450.

Sampath, Prakash, Donlin M. Long, MD, PhD. Henry Brem, MD, The Hunterian Neurosurgical Laboratory: the First Hundred Years of Neurosurgical Research. Neurosurgery, 46 (1) January 2000. pp. 184–95.

Sedalia On–Line. http:www.iland.net/sedalia/about/ (1997).

Semmes, R. Eustace, MD. Walter Dandy, MD, His Relationship to the Society of Neurological Surgeons. Neurosurgery 4, 1979. pp.1 – 2.

Shelton, Mark, Working in a Very Small Place. Vintage Books, New York. !990.

Sparer, Dot. Doctoring In Paradise. Johns Hopkins Medical News, Winter 2000. pp.18–21.

Sylvester, Edward J., The Healing Blade. Beck Press, Tempe Arizona. 1997.

Sugar, O. Dorcas Hager Padget: Artist and Embryologist. Surgical Neurology 38(6), Dec. 1, 1992. pp. 464–468.

Walker, A. Earl. Walter Dandy. The Founders of Neurology. Charles C. Thomas, Springfield, Illinois. 2nd Edition, 1970.

Wilkins, Robert H., Editor, Neurosurgical Classics. American Association of Neurological Surgeons, Johnson Reprints, New York, 1965.

Willard, Adalyn Sands. Letter to Johns Hopkins Hospital Alumnae Magazine, May 1981.

Woodhall, Barnes, MD. Walter Dandy, M.D., Personal Reminiscences. Neurosurgery (4) 1979. pp. 3–6.

Woodhall, Barnes, MD. Neurosurgery in the Past: The Dandy Era. Clinical Neurosurgery Vol. 18, 1971. pp. 1–15.

$\mathcal{P}$hoto Credits

From the Dandy Family Collection: Page 53 (upper photograph). Figures 3.1, 3.2, 3.3, 3.4, 3.5, 3.6, 3.7, 3.8, 3.9, 3.10, 3.11, 3.12,3.14, 3.16, 3.17, 3.18, 3.19, 3.20, 3.21, 3.22, 3.23, 3.24, 3.25, 3.26, 3.27, 3.29, 3.30, 3.31, 3.32, 3.33, 3.34, 3.35, 3.36, 3.37, 3.38, 3.39, 3.41.3.42, 3.43, 3.44, 3.45, 3.46, 3.47, 3.48, 3.49, 3.50, 3.51, 3.52, 3.53, 3.54, 3.55, 3.56, 3.57, 3.58, 3.59, 3.60, 3.61, 3.62, 3.63, 3.64, 3.65, 3.66, 3.67,3.77, 3.83, 3.87, 3.88, 3.89, 3.90, 3.93, 3.97, 3.98, 3.99, 3.101, 3.102, 3.103.

Chapter 4

From Alan Mason Chesney Medical Archives at Johns Hopkins Medical Institutions: Figures 4.1, 4.2, 4.4, 4.5, 4.6, 4.7,4.8, 4.9, 4.10, 4.12, 4.13, 4.14, 4.15, 4.16, 4.16, 4.17, 4.18, 4.19, 4.20, 4.21, 4.22, 4.23, 4.24, 4.28, 4.29, 4.31, 4.32, 4.33, 4.34.
From the Dandy Family Collection: Figures 4.3, 4.11, 4.30.
From North Carolina Collection, University of North Carolina Library at Chapel Hill: Figure 4.25.
From Margaret Mitchell House & Museum: Figure 4.26.
Reprinted courtesy of Joanna T. Steichen: Figure 4.27.

Chapter 5

From the Dandy Family Collection: Figures 5.1, 5.2, 5.3, 5.4, 5.7,5.8, 5.9, 5.10, 5.11, 5.12, 5.13, 5.14.
Courtesy of John Oro', M.D.: Figures 5.5, 5.6.

APPENDIX A

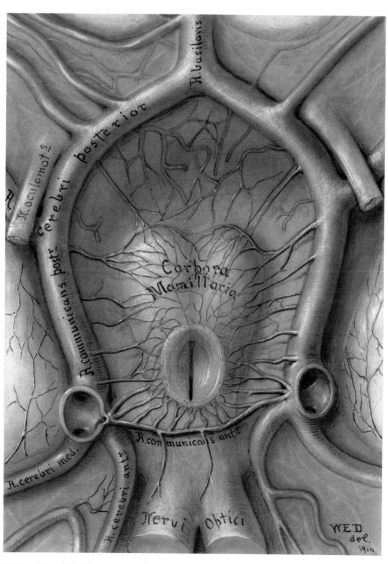

Walter Dandy's illustration of the Blood Supply of the Pituitary Body from
his paper published in 1910–1911.

APPENDIX B

Thomas Wolfe at Johns Hopkins: The Last Days

Walter E. Dandy, Jr., M.D.

The Thomas Wolfe Society invited Dr. Dandy to speak at the Saturday night banquet of our Baltimore meeting to discuss Wolfe's final illness and the treatment he received at Johns Hopkins Hospital. For the 1995 Proceedings, Dr. Dandy provided this written version of his speech:

In her biography of Thomas Wolfe (1960), Elizabeth Nowell noted that I had been an observer in the operating room at Johns Hopkins on September 13, 1938, when Thomas Wolfe was operated on by my father. Although I was only 12 at the time, I had often visited the operating room with my father. I remember well the atmosphere of dejection that followed the operative findings in Wolfe of the untreatable tuberculosis. I have reviewed the records of the operation and its pre-and post-operative course and there is an interesting story related to these records.

As a result of Nowell's mentioning my presence at the operation and of my reading the articles by James Meehan in 1973–74 in which he suggests that Wolfe may have had desert fever (coccidiodomycosis), I had attempted to review these records many years ago. Surprisingly, the Hopkins Record room had no record of Wolfe's hospital stay. This was astonishing, and it wasn't until I read the more recent biography of Wolfe by David Herbert Donald (1987), that I learned that the records had been found in the Houghton Library at Harvard.

This was an extraordinary situation—midical records belong to the hospital of origin, and no notice of transfer or receipt for their removal as found at Johns Hopkins. How Marjorie Fairbanks was able to abscond with the records is still a mystery. In any case, I turned this information over to the Hopkins archives and although the original records were not returned, at least we were sent photocopies. I learned tonight that the ventriculogram X-rays are also in the Houghton Library, having been donated by the late William B. Wisdom of New Orleans.

Ted Mitchell, who guided me through the "Old Kentucky Home" in March, told me that this question of desert fever is still of interest to the Society. In his biography, Donald states that his consultants who reviewed the records were satisfied that tuberculosis was the most likely diagnosis. My father's textbook on brain surgery (1932) refers to an article by C.W. Rand describing coccidioidal granuloma in the spinal cord and brain of two patients. One of these patients was diagnosed as tuberculosis clinically, but at autopsy coccidia were found. These cases occurred in the San Joaquin Valley which is consistent with Meehan's description of Thomas Wolfe's Mojave Desert travel.

161

To compound the mystery in the Hopkins records, the pathological report of the surgical biopsy was reported as showing "non-specific chronic meningitis—there are several small areas composed mostly of macrophages which suggest early tubercle formation, but this appearance is non-specific. The brain itself appears normal. Repeated bacterial and tubercle bacilli stains are negative."

There is confusion in the medical record as to whether the disease found during the operation was miliary tuberculosis or tuberculosis meningitis, or a combination of both. Miliary tuberculosis implies a leakage or showering of tubercle bacilli into the blood stream after rupture of the pulmonary lesion. These bacteria then set up individual granulomas of about the same age and size throughout the body including the brain. The term miliary is derived from the resemblance to millet seeds and from the size (millimeter). Tuberculous meningitis on the other hand, results from a tubercle previously seeded to the brain from the lung, and later ruptured in to the fluid space covering the brain, setting up a infectious reaction. The preoperative diagnosis was most likely tuberculous meningitis, but there was a remote possibility the increased pressure in the brain might have been caused by an expanding but unruptured tubercle obstructing the outflow of spinal fluid. The diagnostic air study made either situation possible. The operative note states that there were myriads of tiny tubercles (miliary) **and** an exudate (meningitis). No large tubercle could be found so that the hydrocephalus had to be due to meningitis.

As an addendum to the above, I spoke last week with Dr. William G. Watson of Pittsburgh, the resident who assisted at the operation. I asked him what he remembered about the operative findings. Although he is now 82 years old, he has no difficulties recalling that it was a "typical case of tuberculous meningitis." Although tuberculosis had not been definitively proven, the evidence that we have is compelling. I wonder whether Meehan had access to hospital records when he postulated his theory of "desert fever."

There are a few points I wold like to make concerning differences and similarities between Wolfe and Dandy. First, I don't believe my father had ever read a novel and had never heard of Thomas Wolfe. On the other hand, he was a voracious reader of biography and history (Churchill, Marlborough, napoleon, and the Civil War and its generals). Fortunately, my mother, who was only three months younger than Wolfe, was able to inform my father of this famous patient. My father somewhat later had another famous novelist as a patient—Margaret Mitchell. Wolfe once described *Gone with the Wind* as an "immortal piece of bilge" and my father never read it. But my father and Mitchell did have a relationship based mutual interest in the civil War. I have a book, *The Army of Tennessee,* that she presented to my father.

Second, I have noticed the many references to Thomas Wolfe's early teachers to whom he was so deeply indebted. Similarly my father frequently commented on several of his early teachers and how underpaid they were. As a result of this influence he never changed a teacher for his services.

I would like now to comment on the last three days of Wolfe's life. The medical records reveal that following his operation he was returned to the neurosurgical recovery room, which we would now call the intensive care unit. During this time notes were taken by the recovery room staff nurses every 15 minutes, including recordings of pulse and respiratory rates, temperatures every hour, intake and output summaries, including fluids by mouth and vein. Interventions such as airway care, including pharyngeal suctioning, urinary catheterization, enemas and ventricular tapping to relieve pressure if necessary, were all documented.

I am bringing this to your attention because it is not generally appreciated that this intensive care unit may have been the first anywhere. It was founded sometime before 1923 by my father. Dr. A.M. Harvey (professor emeritus of medicine, Johns Hopkins

University) has recently published an article documenting this. Harvey notes that the unit was located adjacent to the operating room and close to the doctors' quarters. The three bed unit was staffed 24 hours a day by specially trained nurses. Harvey states, "This was the beginning of careful attention to airway care, temperature control, circulatory monitoring, fluid and electrolyte balance and observation of state of consciousness of the patient. The present surgical intensive care unit of consciousness of the patient. The present surgical intensive care unit is on the site of the earlier unit."

Although this unit did not save Thomas Wolfe's life, it does document the level of his postoperative care, In 1948 I worked one month in this unit and began to appreciate its value. Perhaps that was why I spent the last 16 years of my professional life as full-time director of an intensive care unit. I believe I was the first such person in a community hospital in the United States. (And it was several years before Johns Hopkins had one.)

Finally, I have compared the role of railroads in the life of these two men. Wolfe's writing is full of references to railroading. You may not know the role of railroading in my father's life. He was the son of British immigrants who came to Missouri in the early 1880's to work on the railroads in the developing west. Grandfather Dandy rose to the rank of engineer of the Katy Flyer (the crack train of the MKT). He was an active member of e Brotherhood of Locomotive Engineers (one of the first labor unions) and an ardent Socialist. Wolfe's parents were from a more conservative, perhaps capitalist philosophy, and these influences on their respective sons may have explained some of the differences in their own philosophy. Dandy rejected his parents' Socialist tenets, while Wolfe, for at least part of his life, was definitely interested in Socialist issues.

My father's love for railroading was almost a hobby. As a consultant for the Pennsylvania Railroad, he had a system pass which allowed him to hop a train to Detroit, Chicago, or wherever so that he cold have the seclusion to write his many scientific papers. I accompanied him on several occasions and I also developed an interest in railroading.

I think my father would have appreciated this brief quotation from Wolfe's writings what I found in a recent book on the history of railroads:

> "The rails go westward in the dark
> Have you seen starlight on the rails?
> Have you heard the thunder of the fast express?"

Thank you for coming to Baltimore and thank you for honoring Johns Hopkins and my father.

References

Dandy, Walter E. *Surgery of the Brain.* Baltimore: W.F. Prior Co., Inc. (1932).

Donald, David Herbert. *Look Homeward: A Life of Thomas Wolfe.* Boston: Little Brown (1987).

Harvey, A. McGehee. *Adventures in Medical Research.* Baltimore: Johns Hopkins University Press (1976).

Meehan, James. "How Did Thomas Wolfe Die?" *The State* (September 1973): 18–20, 30.

_____ "Seed of Destruction: The Death of Thomas Wolfe," *South Atlantic Quarterly* 73:2 (Spring 1974): 173–183.

Nowell, Elizabeth. *Thomas Wolfe: A Biography.* Garden City, NY: Double-day & Co. (1960).

Rand, C.W. *Archives of Neurology and Psychiatry* 23 (1930): 8502.

Wolfe, Thomas. *Of Time and the river.* New York: Charles Scribner's Sons (1935): 867.

APPENDIX C

𝒲alter Dandy's Daily Schedule

Excerpt from an article by J. Dewitt Fox. MD.
Walter Dandy–Super-Surgeon. *From Henry Ford Hospital Medical Journal. Vol. 25, No. 3, 1977. pp. 149–170.*

The Dandy day was really a dandy!

Reviewing it will give an insight into the tremendous volume of work Dandy turned out in a day's time as well as the attitudes of some of his residents.

The Dandy service was called "The Brain Team at Hopkins." The last two years of the general surgery residency was spent with Dr. Dandy. He ran the service with dictatorial hand, knowing that the senior years were extremely valuable to each resident in order to complete 8 to 10 years of training.

The resident's daily program had to correlate with Dr. Dandy's. It began several hours before the Chief arrived. So let's take a look at a typical Dandy day at the Hopkins!

6 a.m.—the resident arose and made rounds on the sick patients.

7 a.m.—a quick breakfast when the dinning room opened.

8 a.m.—resident to the operating room. However, no patient could enter the operating room until 8 a.m. because of a longstanding feud with the operating room supervisor. Therefore, it was common practice for the patient to be balanced on the shoulders of the assistant resident and an orderly. At the stroke of 8 a.m., the patient was rushed onto the operating table; the resident began shaving and cleansing the operative area.

Most mornings, several burr holes were placed for ventriculography. Then, the first case was started, which was frequently a posterior approach for a tic or Meniere's syndrome.

9 a.m.—Dr. Dandy arrived and parked by the fire plug in the front of the emergency room.

Dandy would come immediately to the operating room. While he stood in the doorway, the resident would tell him about the sick patients. Unless the patient was a VIP, such as Margaret Mitchell, author of "Gone with the Wind," Dandy never learned the names. Patients were designated as "the man with the frontal lobe tumor from Pittsburgh," or "the lady with the tic from Tallahassee."

165

He would then go to the locker room, put on his operating clothes, while the first case was being opened. Immediately upon section of the nerve, he would place air into one of the burr holes, and drop out. The assistant resident would then take the patient to the x-ray department for ventriculogram films.

Dr. Dandy would view the ventriculogram and appear at the operating room door and state what the next procedure was to be.

The schedule usually contained a brain tumor. A Vth nerve section, an VIIIth nerve section, or a herniated lumbar disc. The schedule always contained from one to three ventriculograms whether or not tumor removals were involved. Since ventriculography originated with Dandy, it was a time-honored procedure, according to Hugo Rizzoli of Washington, D.C. Operations were usually finished by 3 p.m.

4:30 p.m.—his secretary would call and state that Dr. Dandy was on his way to Halsted 7 which was the neurosurgical floor. Complete rounds were made with residents, assistant residents and, frequently, the intern tagging along.

5:30 to 6 p.m.—Dandy was escorted to the emergency room door. He would leave after filching about four cigarettes from the residents or orderly. The residents then returned to the wards to work up the cases and do necessary procedures.

Dandy was partially deaf in his right ear and it was necessary in the halls to walk on his left side, as he spoke in a very low voice and would never repeat himself. The residents had to lean toward him, being careful not to touch him. It was necessary to walk without swinging your right arm and with your head cocked to the right, somewhat like a crab. After a year or more of walking like this, it became a habit. Even to this day, you can recognize Dandy's sold residents by their peculiar crablike gait, reports Dr. Troland.

7 p.m.—The resident on duty always called Dr. Dandy at his home exactly at the stroke of 7 p.m. to report on the condition of the patients and the schedule for the next day's surgery. Sunday nights were an exception; the call had to be made at 7:30 p.m. because Dandy always listened to Jack Benny and would not take any calls during the broadcast.

2 a.m.—Dr. Dandy would frequently want the patients' 2 a.m. temperature reading as well as their 12 midnight ones, so the neurosurgery resident often made night rounds on sick patients. Dandy would frequently call in the middle of the night and ask, "How is the man from Pittsburgh?"

The assistant resident could never talk to Dandy except through the resident. Residents were expected to "work like hell"; many never left the hospital for months at a time.

This rigorous schedule was carried out each day. As tough as it was on residents, Charles Troland, said, "I personally feel that this was an excellent system for teaching. I can only state that I am extremely glad that I had the opportunity to take part in it."

APPENDIX D

The Complete Writings of Walter E. Dandy

I. ARTICLES

1910–1914

1. A human embryo with seven pairs of somites measuring about 2 mm. In length. *Am J Anat* 10:85–108, 1910.

2. The blood supply of the pituitary body. With E. Goetsch. *Am J Anat* 11:137–150, 1910–11.

3. The nerve supply to the pituitary body. *Am J Anat* 15:333–343, 1913.

4. An experimental and clinical study of internal hydrocephalus, with K. D. Blackfan. *JAMA* 61:2216–2217, 1913.

5. Peritoneale und pleurale Resorption in ihren Beziehungen zu der Lagerungebehandlung, with L. G. Rowntree. *Beitr Klin Chir* 87:539–567, 1913.

6. Peritoneal and pleural absorption with reference to postural treatment, with L. G. Rowntree, *Ann Surg* 59:587–596, 1914.

7. Internal hydrocephalus, an experimental, clinical and pathological study, with K. D. Blackfan. *Am J. Dis Child* 8:406–482, 1914.

8. Hydrocephalus internus, eine experimentalle, klinische und pathologische untersuchung, with K. D. Blackfan. *Beitr Klin Chir* 93:392–486, 1914.

9. Zur Kenntnis Der Gutartigen Appendix Tumoren, Speziell *Des Myxoms*. *Beitr Klin Chir* 95:1–7, 1914.

1915–1919

10. Extirpation of the pineal body. *J Exp Med* 22:237–248, 1915.

11. A report of seventy cases of brain tumor, with G. J. Heuer. *Johns Hopkins Hosp Bull* 27:224–237, 1916.

12. Roentgenography in the localization of brain tumor;based upon a series of one hundred consecutive cases, with G. J. Heuer. *Johns Hopkins Hosp Bull* 29:311–322, 1916.

13. Internal hydrocephalus, second paper, with K. D. Blackfan *Am J Dis Child* 14:424–443, 1917.

14. Ventriculography following the injection of air into the cerebral ventricles. *Ann Surg* 68:5–11, 1918.

15. Ventriculography following the injection of air into the cerebral ventricles. *Am J Roentgenol*, n.s., 6:20–26, 1919.

16. Extirpation of the choroids plexus of the lateral ventricles in communicating hydrocephalus. *Ann Surg* 68:560–579, 1918.

17. Fluoroscopy of the cerebral ventricles. *Johns Hopkins Hosp Bull* 30:29–33, 1919.

18. Experimental hydrocephalus. *Ann Surg* 70:129–142, 1919.

19. Pneumoperitoneum: a method of detecting intestinal perforation—an aid in abdominal diagnosis. *Ann Surg* 70:378–384, 1919.

20. Roentgenography of the brain after the injection of air into the spinal canal. *Ann Surg* 70:397–403, 1919.

21. Exhibition of a case of internal hydrocephalus, The Johns Hopkins Medical Society, Jan 21, 1918. *Johns Hopkins Hosp Bull* 29:153–154, 1918.

22. A new hypophysis operation. Devised by G. J. Heuer. Presented by W.E.D. in Heuer's absence. The Johns Hopkins Medical Society, Feb 4, 1918. *Johns Hopkins Hosp Bull* 29:154–155, 1918.

1920–1924

23. Two cases of epilepsy apparently cured by a new form of operative treatment, The Johns Hopkins Medical Society, Feb 16, 1920. *Johns Hopkins Hosp Bull* 31:137–138, 1920.

24. Localization or elimination of cerebral tumors by ventriculography. *Surg Gynecol Obstet* 31:329–342, 1920.

25. The diagnosis and treatment of hydrocephalus resulting from strictures of the aqueduct of Sylvuis. *Surg Gynecol Obstet* 31:340–358, 1920.

26. Hydrocephalus in chondrodystrophy. *Johns Hopkins Hosp Bull* 32:5–8, 1921.

27. The diagnosis and treatment of hydrocephalus due to occlusions of the foramina of Magendie and Luschka. *Surg Gynecol Obstet* 32: 112–124, 1921.

28. The cause of so-called idiopathic hydrocephalus. *Johns Hopkins Hosp Bull* 32:67–75, 1921.

29. An operation for the removal of pineal tumors. *Surg Gynecol Obstet* 33:113–119, 1921

30. The treatment of brain tumors. *JAMA* 77:1853–1859, 1921.

31. Prechiasmal intracranial tumors of the optic nerves. *Am J Ophthalmol* 5:169–188, 1922.

32. Remarks upon certain procedures useful in brain surgery. John Hopkins Hosp Bull 33:188–190, 1922.

   I. Treatment of non-encapsulated brain tumors by extensive resection of contiguous brain tissues.

   II. Diagnosis, localization and removal of tumors of the third ventricle.

   III. Cerebral ventriculoscopy.

   IV. An operation for the removal of large pituitary tumors.

   V. An operative procedure for hydrocephalus.

   VI. Diagnosis and localization of spinal cord tumors.

33. An operation for the total extirpation of tumors in the cerebello-pontine angle: a preliminary report. *Johns Hopkins Hosp Bull* 33: 344–345, 1922.

34. The diagnosis and treatment of brain tumors. *Atlantic Med* J 26:726–728, 1923.

35. A method for the localization of brain tumors in comatose patients: the determination of communication between the cerebral ventricles and the estimation of their position and size without the injection of air (ventricular estimation). *Surg Gynecol Obstet* 36:641–656, 1923.

36. Localization of brain tumors by cerebral pneumography. *Am J Roentgenol* Radium Ther 10:610–612, 1923.

37. The space-compensating function of the cerebrospinal fluid—its connection with cerebral lesions in epilepsy. *Johns Hopkins Hosp Bull* 24:245–251, 1923.

38. Localization of brain tumors by injection of air into the ventricles of the brain. *J Missouri Sate Med Assoc* 21:329–331, 1924.

39. The treatment of staphylococcus and streptococcus meningitis by continuous drainage of the cisterna magna. *Surg Gynecol Obstet* 39:760–774,1924.

1925–1929

40. The diagnosis and localization of spinal cord tumors. *Ann Surg* 81:223–254, 1925.

41. Studies in experimental epilepsy, with Robert Elman. *Bull Johns Hopkins Hosp* 36:40–49, 1925.

42. Section of the sensory root of the trigeminal nerve at the pons: preliminary report of the operative procedure. *Bull Johns Hopkins Hosp* 36:105–106, 1925.

43. Studies on experimental hypophysectomy, L. Effect on the maintenance of life, with F.L. Reichert. *Bull Johns Hopkins Hosp* 37:1–13, 1925.

44. An operation for the total removal of cerebello-pontile (acoustic)tumors. *Surg Gynecol Obstet* 41:129–148, 1925.

45. Intracranial tumors and abscesses causing communicating hydrocephalus. *Ann Surg* 82:199–207, 1925.

46. Contributions to train surgery. A Removal of certain deep-seated brain tumors. B. Intracranial approach with concealed incisions. *Ann Surg* 82:513–525, 1925.

47. Pneumocephalus (intracranial pneumatocele or aerocele). *Arch Surg* 12:949–982, 1926.

48. Ventriculography. *Int Surg Digest* 2:195–198, 1926.

49. Abscesses and inflammatory tumors in the spinal epidural space (so-called pachymeningitis externa). *Arch Surg* 13:477–494, 1926.

50. A sign and symptom of spinal cord tumors. *Arch Neurol Psychiatry* 16:435–441, 1926.

51. Treatment of chronic abscesses of the brain by tapping. *JAMA* 87:1477–1478, 1926.

52. Diagnose und Behandlung der Hirntumoren. *Dtsch Med Wochenschr* 52:638–639, 1926.

53. Experimental investigations on convulsions. *JAMA* 88:90–91, 1927.

54. Impressions of the pathology of epilepsy from operations. *Am J Psychiatry* 6:519–522, 1927.

55. Diagnosis and treatment of brain tumors. NY State J Med 27:285–287, 1927.

56. Glossopharyngeal neuralgia (tic douloureux): its diagnosis and treatment. *Arch Surg* 15:198–214, 1927.

57. Pneumocephalus of bacterial origin. *Arch Surg* 15:913–917, 1927.

58. Removal of right cerebral hemisphere for certain tumors with hemiplegia: preliminary report. *JAMA* 90:823–825, 1928.

59. Méniére's diease: Its diagnosis and a method of treatment. *Arch Surg* 16:1127–1152, 1928.

60. Arteriovenous aneurysms of the brain. *Arch Surg* 17:190–243, 1928.

61. Venous abnormalities and angiomas of the brain. *Arch Surg* 17:715–793, 1928.

62. An operation for the cure of tic douloureux: partial section of the sensory root at the pons. *Arch Surg* 18:687–734, 1929.

63. Where is cerebrospinal fluid absorbed? *JAMA* 92:2012–2014, 1929.

64. Operative relief from pain in lesions of the mouth, tongue and throat. *Arch Surg* 19:143–148, 1929.

65. An operative treatment for certain cases of meningocele (or encephalocele) into the orbit. *Arch Ophthalmol* 2:123–132, 1929.

66. Mechanisms and symptoms of tumors of the third ventricle and pineal body. *Intracranial Pressure in Health and Disease*, vol 8 of a Series of Research Publications, Association for Research in Nervous and Mental Diseases. Baltimore, Williams & Wilkins, 1929, pp 375–385.

67. Loose cartilage from intervertebral disk simulating tumor of the spinal cord. *Arch Surg* 19:660–672, 1929.

1930–1934

68. Injuries to the head. J Med Soc NJ 27:91–97, 1930. Also in the *Int J Med Surg* 43:237–242, 1930.

69. An operation for the treatment of spasmodic torticollis. *Arch Surg* 20:1021–1032, 1930.

70. Changes in our conceptions of localization of certain functions in the brain. *Am J Physiol.* 93:643, 1930.

71. The course of the nerve fibers transmitting sensation of taste, with Dean Lewis. *Arch Surg* 21:249–288, 1930.

72. Skull, brain and its membranes. In Graham EA (ed): *Surgical Diagnosis: By American Authors.* Philadelphia, WB Saunders, 1930, vol III, pp 846–898.

73. Congenital cerebral cysts of the cavum septi pellucidi (fifth ventricle) and cavum vergae (sixth ventricle): diagnosis and treatment. *Arch Neurol Psychiatry* 25:44–66, 1931.

74. "Avertin" anesthesia in neurologic surgery, *JAMA* 96:1860–1862, 1931.

75. Treatment of hemicrania (migraine) by removal of the inferior cervical and first thoracic sympathetic ganglion. *Bull Johns Hopkins Hosp* 48:357–361, 1931.

76. Epilepsy. Read the Annual Meeting of Medical and Surgical Section, American Railway Association, New York City, June 8, 1931, and published in the *Proceedings* of the Association in the Fall 1931, pp 3–12.

77. Diagnosis and treatment of lesions of the cranial nerves. *Bull Assoc Surg Missouri Pacific Railway.* January, 1932.

78. Certain functions of the roots and ganglia of the cranial sensory nerves. *Arch Neurol Psychiatry* 27:22–26, 1932.

79. The importance of more adequate sterilization processes in hospitals. *Bull Am Coll Surg* 16:11–12, 1932.

80. Effect of total removal of left temporal lobe in a right-handed person: localization of areas of brain concerned with speech. *Arch Neurol Psychiatry* 27:221–224, 1932.

81. The treatment of trigeminal neuralgia by the cerebellar route. *Ann Surg* 96:787–795, 1932.

82. The diagnosis and treatment of Méniére's disease. *Trans Am Ther Soc* for 1932, pp 128–130.

83. Méniére's disease: diagnosis and treatment: report of thirty cases. *Am J Surg*, o.s., 20:693–698, 1933.

84. Physiological studies following extirpation of the right cerebral hemisphere in man. *Bull Johns Hopkins Hosp* 53:31–51, 1933.

85. Treatment of Méniére's disease by section of only the vestibular portion of the acoustic nerve. *Bull Johns Hopkins Hosp* 53:52–55, 1933.

86. Diagnosis and treatment of injuries of the head. *JAMA* 101:772–775, 1933.

87. Benign encapsulated tumors in the lateral ventricles of the brain: diagnosis and treatment. *Ann Surg* 98:841–845, 1933.

88. Cerebral (ventricular) hydrodynamic test for thrombosis of the lateral sinus. *Arch Otolaryngol* 19:297–302, 1934.

89. The diagnosis and treatment of lesions of the cranial nerves. *Del State Med J* 6:153–160, 1934.

90. Concerning the cause of trigeminal neuralgia. *Am J Surg*, n.s., 24:447–455, 1934.

91. The effect of hemisection of the cochlear ranch of the human auditory nerve. Preliminary report. *Bull Johns Hopkins Hosp* 54:208–210, 1934.

92. Méniére's disease: symptoms, objective findings and treatment in forty-two cases. *Arch Otolaryngol* 20:1–30, 1934.

93. Removal of cerebellopontile (acoustic) tumors through a unilateral approach. *Arch Surg* 29:337–344, 1934.

94. The treatment of so-called pseudo-Méniére's disease. *Bull Johns Hopkins Hosp* 55:232–239, 1934.

95. Effects on hearing after subtotal section of the cochlear branch of the auditory nerve. *Bull Johns Hopkins Hosp* 55:240–243, 1934.

1935–1939

96. The treatment of intracranial hemorrhage resulting from cisternal puncture. *Bull Johns Hopkins Hosp* 56:294–301, 1935.

97. The treatment of carotid cavernous arteriovenous aneurysms. *Ann Surg* 102:916–920, 1935.

98. The treatment of bilateral Méniére's disease and pseudo-Méniére's disease. *Trans Am Neurol Assoc* 61:128–133, 1935; also in *Acta Neuropathol* in honorem Ludovici Puusepp, Tartu, Estonia, *Folia Neuropathol Estoniana* 60:10–14, 1935.

99. Polyuria and polydipsia (diabetes insipidus) and glycosuria resulting from animal experiments on the hypophysis and its environs, with F. L. Reichert, *Bull Johns Hopkins Hosp* 58:418–427, 1936.

100. The treatment of injuries of the head. *Pennsylvania Med J* 39:755–759, 1936.

101. Operative experience in cases of pineal tumor. *Arch Surg* 33:19–46, 1936.

102. [The treatment of carotid cavernous aneurysms, pulsating exophthalmos.] *Soviet Surg* 2:736–739, 1936 (in Russian).

103. Carotid-cavernous aneurysms (pulsating exophthalmos). *Zentralbl Neurochir Z Jahrgang*, N.R. 2:77–113, 1937: N.R. 3:165–206. Also *Int J Neurol Contrib*, Prof. Wilhelm Tönnis, Wurzburg, Germany.

104. Pathological changes in Méniére's disease. *JAMA* 108:931–937, 1937.

105. Méniére's disease: its diagnosis and treatment. *South Med J* 30:621–623, 1937.

106. Etiological and clinical types of so-called nerve deafness. *Laryngoscope* 47:594–597, 1937.

107. Diagnosis and treatment of brain tumors. *Alabama Med Assoc J* 6:162–166, 1936; also *Ohio State Med J* 33:17–18, 1937.

108. Brain tumors. Texas State J Med 32:833, 1937.

109. Injuries of the head, *Proceedings of the Seventeenth Annual Meeting of the Medical and Surgical Section of the Association of American Railroads*, June 7–8, 1937, pp 96–105.

110. Intracranial pressure without brain tumor. *Ann Surg* 106:492–513, 1937.

111. Diagnosis and treatment of brain abscess. *Proceedings of the Inter-State Post Graduate Medical Assembly of North America*, 1937, pp 235–238.

112. Studies on experimental hypophysectomy in dogs: III. Somatic, mental and glandular effects, with F. L. Reichert. *Bull Johns Hopkins Hosp* 62:122–155, 1938.

113. Intracranial aneurysm of the internal carotid artery cured by operation. *Ann Surg* 107:654–659, 1938.

114. Diagnosis and treatment of lesions of the cranial nerves. *Rocky Mt Med J* 35:282–288, 1938.

115. The operative treatment of communicating hydrocephalus. *Ann Surg* 108:194–202, 1938.

116. Trigeminal neuralgia and pains in the face. *J Indiana State Med Assoc* 31:669–672, 1938.

117. The surgery of Méniére's disease. In Kipetzky SJ (ed): *Surgery of the Ear, Nelson's Loose-Leaf Surgery of the Ear*. New York and Edinburgh, Thomas Nelson's and Sons, 1938 and 1946, ch 16, pp 387–398.

118. Subdural hematoma: diagnosis and treatment, with P. A. Kunkel. *Ann Surg* 38:24–54, 1939.

119. The treatment of internal carotid aneurysms within the cavernous sinus and the cranial chamber: report of three cases. *Ann Surg* 109:689–709, 1939.

120. Papilloedema without intracranial pressure (optic neuritis). *Ann Surg* 110:161–168, 1939.

121. The central connections of the vestibular pathways: an experimental study, with P. A. Kunkel. *Am J Med Sci* 198:149–155, 1939.

122. Lesions of the cranial nerves: diagnosis and treatment. *J Ins Coll Surg* 2:5–14, 1939.

123. Intracranial aneurysms, *Proceedings of the Third Congress of the Pan-Pacific Surgical Association*, Honolulu, Hawaii, September 15–21, 1939, pp 335–336.

124. Méniére's disease, *Proceedings of the Third Congress of the Pan-Pacific Surgical Association,* Honolulu, Hawaii, September 15–21, 1939. pp 357–364.

1940–1946

125. Section of the human hypophyseal stalk: its relation to diabetes insipidus and hyphpseal functions. *JAMA* 114:312–314, 1940.

126. On the relationship of dentistry to certain neurological diseases (Paper given at the Dental Centenary Celebration, Baltimore, March 18, 1940). *Proceedings of the Dental Centenary Celebration,* March, 1940, Sponsors: Maryland State Dental Association and American Dental Association, pp 140–144.

127. Removal of longitudinal sinus *involved* in tumors. *Arch Surg* 41:244–256, 1940.

128. The surgical treatment of Méniére's disease (Presented before the Clinical Congress of the American College of Surgeons, Chicago, October 21–25, 1940). *Surg Gynecol Obstet* 72:421–425, 1941.

129. Results following the transcranial operative attack on orbital tumors. *Arch Ophthalmol* 25:191–213, 1941.

130. On the pathology of carotid-cavernous aneurysms (pulsating exophthalmos), with R. H. Follis, Jr. *Am J Ophthalmol* 24:365–385, 1941.

131. The surgical treatment of intracranial aneurysms of the internal carotid artery. *Ann Surg* 114:336–339, 1941.

132. Concealed ruptured intervertebral disks: a plea for the elimination of contrast media in diagnosis. *JAMA* 117:821–823, 1941.

133. Recent advances in the diagnosis and treatment of ruptured intervertebral disks. *Ann Surg* 115:514–520, 1942.

134. Serious complications of ruptured intervertebral disks. *JAMA* 119:474–477, 1942.

135. Aneurysm of the anterior cerebral artery. *JAMA* 119:1253–1254, 1942.

136. Improved localization and treatment of ruptured intervertebral disks. *JAMA* 120:605–607, 1942.

137. Intracranial arterial aneurysms in the carotid canal. *Arch Surg* 45:335–350, 1942.

138. Results following ligation of the internal carotid artery. *Arch Surg* 45:521–533, 1942.

139. A method of restoring nerves requiring resection. *JAMA* 122:35–36, 1943.

140. An operation for scaphocephaly. *Arch Surg* 47:247–249, 1943.

141. Recent advances in the treatment of ruptured (lumbar) intervertebral disks. *Ann Surg* 118:639–646, 1943.

142. The treatment of essential hypertension by sympathectomy: a report on twelve patients three to seven years following operation. With James Bordley, III and Morton Galdston. *Bull Johns Hopkins Hosp* 72:127–165, 1943.

143. Newer aspects of ruptured intervertebral disks. *Ann Surg* 119:481–484, 1944.

144. A procedure to correct facial paralysis, with Edward M. Hanrahan. *JAMA* 124:1051–1053, 1944.

145. Pathogenesis of intermittent exophthalmos, with Frank B. Walsh. *Arch Ophthalmol* 32:1–10, 1944.

146. Treatment of rhimorrhea and otorrhea. *Arch Surg* 49:75–85, 1944.

147. Treatment of recurring attacks of low backache without sciatica. *JAMA* 125:1175–1178, 1944.

148. Electroencephalograms taken at the Henry Phipps Psychiatric Clinic on One Hundred Patients on the Neurological Service, The Johns Hopkins Hospital, Baltimore, 1938–1940, pp 51–63.

149. Treatment of aneurysms of the brain. *Proceedings of the Twentieth Annual Meeting of the Medical and Surgical Section of the Association of American Railroads,* June 10–11, 1940, pp 51–63.

150. Results of removal of acoustic tumors by the unilateral approach. *Arch Surg* 42:1026–1033, 1944

151. Diagnosis and treatment of lesions of the cranial nerves. *J Med* 22:239–245, 1941.

152. The diagnosis and treatment of ruptured intervertebral disks. *The Medical Comment*, Johnstown, Pennsylvania, 26:4–7, 17, July, 1944.

153. Recent advances in the diagnosis and treatment of ruptured intervertebral disks. *Neuracirugia*, Santiago, Chile, 2 (Anos 1941–1943), 1944, 4 pp.

154. The treatment of spondylolistheses. *JAMA* 127:137–139, 1945.

155. Méniére's disease in a deaf-mute. *Arch Surg* 50:74–76, 1945.

156. Diagnosis and treatment of strictures of the aqueduct of Sylvius (causing hydrocephalus). *Arch Surg* 51:1–14, 1945.

157. Arteriovenous aneurysms of the scalp and face. *Arch Surg* 52:1–32, 1946.

158. Results following bands and ligatures on the human internal carotid artery. *Ann Surg* 123:384–396, 1946.

159. The treatment of an unusual subdural hydroma (external hydrocephalus). *Arch Surg* 52:421–428, 1946.

160. The location of the conscious center in the brain—the corpus striatum. *Bull Johns Hopkins Hosp* 79:34–58, 1946.

II. BOOKS

1. Surgery of the brain. In: Lewis D (ed): *Practice of Surgery*. Hagerstown, MD, WF Prior, 1932, vol 12, ch 1.

2. *Benign Tumors in the Third Ventricle of the Brain: Diagnosis and Treatment*. Springfield, IL Charles C. Thomas, 1933.171 pp.

3. *Benign, Encapsulated Tumors in the Lateral Ventricles of the Brain: Diagnosis and Treatment*. Baltimore, Williams & Wilkins, 1934, 189 pp.

4. *Orbital Tumors: Results Following the Transcranial Operative Attack*. New York, Oskar Piest, 1941, xv, 168 pp.

5. *Intracranial Arterial Aneurysms*. Ithaca, NY, Comstock Publishing Company, Cornell University, 1944, viii, 147 pp.

6. *Surgery of the Brain* (A monograph from Volume 12 of *Lewis' Practice of Surgery*). Hagerstown, MD, WF Prior, 1945, 671 pp.

7. *Selected Writings of Walter E Dandy*. Compiled by Charles E. Trolund and Frank J. Otenasek. Springfield, IL, Charles C. Thomas, 1957, vii, 789 pp.

8. *The Brain*. Hagerstown, MD, WF Prior, 1966, 671 pp.

Name Index

Subject Index